Epilepsy in Women

Epilepsy in Women

EDITED BY

Cynthia L. Harden MD

Professor of Neurology
Chief, Division of Epilepsy and Electroencephalography
Hofstra North Shore-LIJ School of Medicine
Cushing Neuroscience Institutes, Brain and Spine Specialists
North Shore-Long Island Jewish Health System
Great Neck, New York
USA

Sanjeev V. Thomas MD, DM

Professor of Neurology
Department of Neurology
Sree Chitra Tirunal Institute for Medical Sciences and Technology
Trivandrum, Kerala State
India

Torbjörn Tomson MD, PhD

Professor of Neurology and Epileptology
Karolinska Institutet
Stockholm
Sweden

WILEY-BLACKWELL

A John Wiley & Sons, Ltd., Publication

Registered Office
John Wiley & Sons, Ltd, The Atrium, Southern Gate, Chichester, West Sussex, PO19 8SQ, UK

Editorial Offices
9600 Garsington Road, Oxford, OX4 2DQ, UK
The Atrium, Southern Gate, Chichester, West Sussex, PO19 8SQ, UK
111 River Street, Hoboken, NJ 07030-5774, USA

For details of our global editorial offices, for customer services and for information about how to apply for permission to reuse the copyright material in this book please see our website at www.wiley.com/wiley-blackwell

Library of Congress Cataloging-in-Publication Data

Epilepsy in women / edited by Cynthia L. Harden, Sanjeev V. Thomas, Torbjörn Tomson.
  p. ; cm.
  Includes bibliographical references and index.
  ISBN 978-0-470-67267-9 (hardback : alk. paper)
I. Harden, Cynthia L.   II. Thomas, Sanjeev V.   III. Tomson, Torbjörn, 1950–
[DNLM: 1. Epilepsy–etiology.   2. Epilepsy–physiopathology.   3. Menstruation–
physiology.   4. Pregnancy Complications.   5. Sex Factors.   6. Women's Health. WL 385]
  616.85′30082–dc23
                                                          2012037052

A catalogue record for this book is available from the British Library.

Cover image: ©iStockphoto/billyfoto
Cover design by Meaden Creative

Set in 9.5/13pt Meridien by SPi Publisher Services, Pondicherry, India
Printed and bound in Singapore by Markono Print Media Pte Ltd

1   2013

Contents

Preface

The science and practice of caring for women with epilepsy is constantly evolving and progressing. The relative teratogenic risks of specific anti-epileptic drugs (AEDs), the nuances of monitoring AED levels during pregnancy and the capacity for epilepsy itself to be an endocrine disruptor are important findings that have changed practice, even as the field continues to be explored and refined. The editors present a comprehensive current snapshot of issues for women with epilepsy, couched around a clinical case relevant to each chapter which they hope will strike readers as both familiar and illuminating. While research is ongoing, this book comes at a time when some scientific milestones in the field have been reached. It can be confidently presented, for example, that multiple worldwide registries on pregnancy outcomes of women with epilepsy are consistent in their findings of implicating valproate as having a dose-related risk for both structural and cognitive teratogenesis with a risk above other AEDs. The complexity of contraceptive management is also now abundantly clear, and the expert recommendation is a simplified approach of avoiding hormonal contraceptives for women taking cytochrome P450 enzyme-inducing AEDs. With regard to the many unanswered questions in the field, this book aims to inform the reader about ongoing research avenues such as mechanisms of AED teratogenesis, reproductive hormonal neurophysiologic effects, and psychological risks for women with epilepsy, to cite several, in order to provide an update and a solid background to inform emerging clinical guidance. Linking epilepsy to other areas of neurology, with a recognition that neurologic illness cannot be as compartmentalized as perhaps we would like it to be, the editors have included an important clinical chapter discussing the differential diagnosis and evaluation for new-onset seizures during pregnancy.

It is intended that the joy and enthusiasm the editors have for the science of this field, for the wonderful patients we have had the privilege to care for, and for educating others are evident in this book. Our greatest emotion, however, is gratitude to the contributors, who have graciously shared their insight and expertise in chapters that are always enlightening and often downright poetic. The roster of contributors is an amazing group of international leaders distinguished by their scientific rigor combined with creativity, evident in the chapters written by each. The editors hope that the reader will enjoy each chapter and find them useful and thought-provoking, as well as discovering tenets that are timeless in an ever-changing field.

Cynthia L. Harden
Sanjeev V. Thomas
Torbjörn Tomson

Contributors

Dina Battino MD
Epilepsy Centre, Department of
Neurophysiology and Experimental
Epileptology
IRCCS (Istituto di Ricovero a Cura a Carattere
Scientifico) Neurological Institute "Carlo Besta"
Foundation
Milan, Italy

Ettore Beghi MD
Head of Laboratory of Neurological Disorders
Istituto di Ricerche Farmacologiche
"Mario Negri"
Milano, Italy

Massimiliano Beghi MD
Dipartimento di Salute Mentale
Ospedale "G. Salvini"
Garbagnate Milanese, Italy

Ingrid Borthen MD, PhD
Senior Consultant
Head of the Obsterical Department
Haukeland University Hospital
Bergen, Norway

Lynsey E. Bruce MS
Dell Pediatric Research Institute
Department of Nutritional Sciences
University of Texas at Austin
Austin, Texas
USA

Anne R. Davis MD, MPH
Associate Professor of Clinical Obstetrics and
Gynecology
Department of Obstetrics and Gynecology
Columbia University Medical Center
New York, New York
USA

Richard H. Finnell PhD
Professor, Dell Pediatric Research Institute
Departments of Nutritional Sciences, Chemistry
and Biochemistry
University of Texas at Austin;
Director, Genomic Research
Dell Children's Medical Center
Austin, Texas
USA

Peter B. Forgacs MD
Rockefeller University
New York, New York
USA

Evan R. Gedzelman MD
Assistant Director of Clinical Neurophysiology
Fellowship with Epilepsy Focus
Assistant Professor of Neurology
Emory University School of Medicine
Department of Neurology
Atlanta, Georgia
USA

Nils Erik Gilhus MD, PhD
Professor of Neurology, Department of Clinical
Medicine, University of Bergen
Senior Consultant in Neurology
Haukeland University Hospital
Bergen, Norway

Cynthia L. Harden MD
Professor of Neurology
Chief, Division of Epilepsy and
Electroencephalography
Hofstra North Shore-LIJ School of Medicine
Cushing Neuroscience Institutes, Brain and
Spine Specialists
North Shore-Long Island Jewish Health System
Great Neck, New York
USA

Vilho K. Hiilesmaa MD, PhD
Department of Obstetrics and Gynecology
Helsinki University Central Hospital
Helsinki, Finland

Usha Kini MBBS, MRCP, FRCP, MD
Consultant Clinical Geneticist and Honorary
Senior Lecturer University of Oxford
Department of Clinical Genetics
Oxford University Hospitals NHS Trust
Oxford, UK

Autumn M. Klein MD, PhD
Chief, Division of Women's Neurology
Assistant Professor of Neurology and Obstetrics
and Gynecology
Departments of Neurology and Obstetrics and
Gynecology
UPMC Presbyterian/Magee Women's Hospital
of UPMC
Pittsburgh, Pennsylvania
USA

Gerhard Luef MD
Associate Professor in Neurology
Head of the Epilepsy Study Group
Department of Neurology
Medical University Innsbruck
Innsbruck, Austria

Kimford J. Meador MD
Director of the Emory Epilepsy Center
Professor of Neurology
Emory University School of Medicine
Department of Neurology
Atlanta, Georgia
USA

Kathleen M. Morrell MD
Assistant Clinical Professor of Obstetrics and
Gynecology
Department of Obstetrics and
Gynecology
Columbia University Medical Center
New York, New York
USA

Aparna Nair PhD
Assistant Professor
Centre for Development Studies
Trivandrum
Kerala, India

Alison M. Pack MD, MPH
Associate Professor of Clinical Neurology
Department of Neurology
Neurological Institute of New York
Columbia University Medical Center
New York, New York
USA

Ana M. Palacios MD
Dell Pediatric Research Institute
Department of Nutritional Sciences
University of Texas at Austin
Austin, Texas
USA

Page B. Pennell MD
Associate Professor in Neurology
Director of Research, Division of Epilepsy
Harvard Medical School
Brigham and Women's Hospital
Boston, Massachusetts
USA

Doodipala Samba Reddy PhD, RPh
Associate Professor
Department of Neuroscience and Experimental
Therapeutics
College of Medicine
Texas A&M Health Science Center
Bryan, Texas
USA

Line S. Røste MD, PhD
Senior Consultant
Department of Neurology
Oslo University Hospital – Rikshospitalet
Oslo, Norway

Anne Sabers MD, DMSc
Epilepsy Clinic
Department of Neurology
University State Hospital – Rigshospitalet
Copenhagen, Denmark

Sigrid Svalheim MD, PhD
Senior Consultant
Department of Neurology
Oslo University Hospital – Rikshospitalet
Oslo, Norway

Erik Taubøll MD, PhD
Professor of Neurology and Section Head
Department of Neurology
Oslo University Hospital – Rikshospitalet
Oslo, Norway

Kari A. Teramo MD, PhD
Department of Obstetrics and Gynecology
Helsinki University Central Hospital
Helsinki, Finland

Sanjeev V. Thomas MD, DM
Professor of Neurology
Department of Neurology
Sree Chitra Tirunal Institute for Medical
Sciences and Technology
Trivandrum
Kerala, India

Torbjörn Tomson MD, PhD
Professor of Neurology and Epileptology
Department of Clinical Neuroscience
Karolinska Institutet
Stockholm, Sweden

Bogdan J. Wlodarczyk
Assistant Professor
Dell Pediatric Research Institute
Department of Nutritional Sciences
University of Texas at Austin
Austin, Texas
USA

CHAPTER 1

Gender Difference in Epidemiology and Comorbidities of Epilepsy

Ettore Beghi[1] and Massimiliano Beghi[2]

[1]Laboratorio di Malattie Neurologiche, Istituto di Ricerche Farmacologiche "Mario Negri", Milano, Italy

[2]Dipartimento di Salute Mentale, Ospedale "G. Salvini", Garbagnate Milanese, Italy

> **Case history:** *A 54-year-old woman with multiple sclerosis was first seen at an epilepsy center seeking expert advice after having received a diagnosis of post-traumatic epilepsy by her general practitioner. At age 16 years the patient was a victim of a car accident during which she was seriously injured in her head. A temporo-occipital subdural hematoma was evacuated with uneventful follow-up. At that time, the patient received prophylactic treatment with phenytoin for 6 months. At age 30, she had blurring of vision for 3 weeks and at age 35 she had numbness in her left leg associated with mild weakness and urinary urgency. A diagnosis of multiple sclerosis was made based on history, clinical findings, and MRI evidence of demyelinating disease. Neurological symptoms and signs disappeared 1 month after onset and recurred, but with lower severity and duration, at age 45. In the 3 months preceding the epilepsy consultation, the patient experienced episodes characterized by visual hallucinations, each lasting 1–2 min. A follow-up MRI showed multiple areas of increased intensity with periventricular distribution in the frontal and occipital areas. The following questions were posed by the patient to the epileptologist. (1) Is this epilepsy or simply a relapse of her multiple sclerosis? (2) Is head trauma the most plausible cause of her seizures? (3) Should antiepileptic treatment be taken for life?*

Background and important detail

The frequency, etiology, and prognosis of epilepsy in men and women can be better outlined through population-based epidemiological studies. The diagnosis of epilepsy is made by epidemiologists when the patient experiences at least two unprovoked seizures 24 or more hours apart [1]. This definition has been revised by the International League Against

Epilepsy in Women, First Edition. Edited by Cynthia L. Harden, Sanjeev V. Thomas and Torbjörn Tomson.

Epilepsy and the International Bureau for Epilepsy [2] which suggested that epilepsy can be predicted by a single seizure. However, the revision is not likely to affect gender-specific epidemiological indices, because there is no evidence that men and women have a different risk of relapse after a first unprovoked seizure.

Patients with epilepsy enrolled in epidemiological studies should represent the entire spectrum of the disease. Population-based surveys have been conducted in patients with epilepsy of all ages or in selected age groups (children, adults, elderly). In these studies, men and women were often compared. Several studies, especially those from developing countries, have been performed only in patients with major seizures. Others were limited to selected seizure types or epilepsy syndromes. Most surveys have been conducted in small urban or rural areas, with no nationally based reports and no international comparisons [3]. The sociocultural background of the underlying population (which has significant effects on the frequency and characteristics of the disease) may be a strong confounder when different populations are compared. This is particularly true when men and women are compared. Patients with mild or infrequent seizures may not receive medical care. Patients may also deny a history of epilepsy for fear of being stigmatized. This is particularly true in less developed countries where women are more likely than men to conceal the disease. In addition, in community surveys it may be difficult to exclude psychogenic nonepileptic seizures, which may occur in up to one-fourth of patients presenting to family physicians [4] and tend to prevail in women, who may account for about three-fourths of reported cases of such nonepileptic seizures [5]. Although community-based studies including all forms of epilepsy provide a better view of the whole spectrum of the disease, studies in patients with selected epileptogenic conditions may demonstrate different rates of occurrence in men and women because of differences in the gender distribution of the underlying disease.

Other methodological constraints and inconsistencies, in terms of case ascertainment and study conduct, may be present in studies performed in developing countries [6]. The quality and completeness of data collection is impaired by the use of standard screening instruments across populations with diverse social and cultural backgrounds (with different effects in men and women), the lack of specialized personnel, the virtual lack of diagnostic equipment, and the use of different terminologies to define seizures and epilepsy.

Incidence of epilepsy

With few exceptions [7–9], the incidence of epilepsy and unprovoked seizures is higher in men than in women in both industrialized and developing countries, although the difference is not significant in the large majority of reports. In a recent Finnish survey, the incidence remained slightly higher [relative risk (RR) 1.21, 95% confidence interval (CI) 1.19–1.23] in men than women in all age groups and all regions and throughout the entire observation period [10]. However, the risk of developing epilepsy differs between men and women according to age. In a white population in the USA, the 50-year age-specific annual incidence of epilepsy was similar in the two sexes until about 50 years of age and was significantly higher in older men than in women [11]. In men, the cumulative incidence rate was 0.42% at age 65–69, 0.85% at age 70–74, 1.84% at age 75–79, 2.40% at age 80–84, 3.75% at age 85–89 and 4.26% at age 90 and older. The corresponding rates in women were 0.24, 0.52, 0.94, 1.53, 2.24, and 2.77%.

In the Icelandic population [12], the age-specific incidence was similar in male and female patients up to age 85 and older, when the incidence in women was half that in men. The results were similar in studies carried out in Switzerland and Estonia [3]. Studies done in children and adolescents reported incidences of 41–82 per 100 000 per year, with rates 30–60% higher in girls before the age of 5 years and 10–20% higher in boys in later childhood and adolescence [13]. These differences may be explained by the differing distribution of factors known to increase risk of epilepsy in children. These include congenital malformations of the central nervous system (CNS), moderate or severe head trauma, CNS infections, certain inherited metabolic conditions, and genetic factors. However, these differences can also be explained by factors intrinsic to the study populations and the methods of case ascertainment.

Prevalence of epilepsy

As with incidence, the prevalence of epilepsy is higher in men than in women. Among population-based studies in Europe [3], all but one [14] found higher prevalence ratios in males than females. However, the difference was only rarely statistically significant [15–18] and, in most studies, sex dominance shifted between age groups. In children, the prevalence was slightly higher in boys than in girls [13].

The distribution of epilepsy in men and women has been shown to vary across countries. This can be mostly explained by the same factors discussed with incidence. These include differences in genetic background, the prevalence of the commonest risk factors, the concealment of the disease by women for sociocultural reasons, and perhaps the structure of the study population and the methods of case ascertainment.

Epilepsy syndromes and comorbidity

Epilepsy is a heterogeneous clinical condition characterized by differing syndromic patterns. Absence seizures are reported to be more common in girls than in boys, while both infantile spasms and Lennox–Gastaut syndrome are more common in males than in females [13]. Juvenile myoclonic epilepsy and other epilepsies of adolescence have an equal distribution between boys and girls [19]. Although in clinical series some epilepsy syndromes have been found to prevail in boys and others in girls, with few exceptions these observations have been rarely confirmed by community-based studies. In a white population in the USA, symptomatic partial epilepsies have been found to prevail in women and nonlocalized cryptogenic partial epilepsies in men, although gender-specific incidence rates were not available [20]. A community-based survey carried out in Croatia found that more males than females had generalized seizures, whereas more females than males had partial seizures [21].

The association between epilepsy and an epileptogenic condition (e.g., head trauma) does not necessarily establish a cause-and-effect relationship. In order for a given variable to be considered a risk factor for epilepsy, a number of conditions must be satisfied, including temporal relationship, strength, consistency, biological gradient, and biological plausibility of the association [22]. Cerebrovascular disorders, head trauma, developmental disorders, and CNS infection are the most common etiological factors in well-defined populations. However, using for reference the frequency of epilepsy in the general population, the clinical conditions carrying the highest risk of seizures and epilepsy are, in decreasing order, cerebral palsy (RR 17.9–34.4), mental retardation (RR 22.6–31), stroke (RR 22), CNS infections (RR 10.8), and multiple sclerosis (RR 3.6) [23]. Severe traumatic brain injury carries a 17-fold risk of seizures [24]. However, the risk decreases over time and overlaps that of the general population after 20 years. This is also true for other acute CNS insults while a high risk of seizures and epilepsy may persist with time in chronic or relapsing clinical conditions.

No gender differences were found between epilepsy and severe handicap in children with temporal lobe epilepsy followed up for 20 years [25]. In the general population, learning disorders are more common in boys than in girls (odds ratio, OR, 1.4–3.2) [26] and are present in up to one-fourth of patients with epilepsy [27] with no robust indication of a gender difference.

Migraine [28], attention-deficit hyperactivity disorder (ADHD) [29], and several psychiatric illnesses [30] have differing distribution in men and women. In these clinical conditions the risk of seizures and epilepsy is higher than expected and may affect men and women to a differing extent. Although the results of published reports are inconsistent, comorbidity can be interpreted in light of a common genetic susceptibility and/or the presence of shared environmental factors. In a cross-sectional population-based study extracting data from the UK General Practice Research Database, psychiatric disorders occurred twice as often in people with epilepsy compared with the rest of the population, with significant differences between sexes (rate ratio 2.36 in men and 1.87 in women, with the largest differences for anxiety and depression) [30]. In this population, the risk of migraine was also increased, with a significant difference between men and women (rate ratio 2.22 vs. 1.44). In the Canadian Community Health Survey, a population-based prevalence study of several psychiatric conditions associated with epilepsy, major depressive disorder had a statistically significant age-by-sex interaction such that the sex difference (women>men) was seen to decline with age [31].

Clear-cut gender differences related to the etiology and comorbidity of epilepsy are difficult to find because the exact attribution of cause is often not possible and because a number of factors are likely to be involved in causation in a single individual.

A population-based study carried out in Norway showed that girls with epilepsy did not exhibit risk-taking behaviors (daily alcohol consumption, illegal drug use, criminal offences) more frequently than controls, but having epilepsy was a risk factor for such behavior in boys (OR 3.2) [32,33]; girls had more emotional problems, whereas boys had higher scores regarding peer relationship and hyperactivity/inattention problems. Male gender, low socioeconomic status (family income below poverty limit and living with a single parent), and other chronic diseases (asthma/diabetes) were independent risk factors for developing psychiatric symptoms, along with epilepsy. However, having or having had epilepsy was a much stronger risk factor for developing psychiatric symptoms in girls than in boys (OR 4.2 vs. 2.3). This finding is in line with other reports [34–36] but in contrast with others [37–40].

Attitudes toward epilepsy and gender

Sociocultural factors may play a major role in affecting differing public attitudes toward epilepsy in men and women. In India, a survey performed in a tertiary center in patients with juvenile myoclonic epilepsy and temporal lobe epilepsy indicated that comorbidities, lower employment, and higher anxiety state were more frequent for women than for men. Compared with men, women had more difficulty finding life partners, were at increased risk of divorce, and had more problems with employment, even when the clinical profiles of their epilepsy syndromes were comparable [40]. However, these results were not confirmed in other studies [42–45] or could be verified only in selected patient subgroups (e.g., more unemployed women among those married) [46].

Prognosis and mortality of epilepsy

Population studies in western countries in patients with newly diagnosed epilepsy followed for several decades show that up to 80% of cases enter prolonged periods of seizure remission and up to 50% continue to be seizure-free after treatment discontinuation (terminal remission) [47,48]. The probability of long-term remission is similar in men and women and differences, where present, remain small when treatment is discontinued. These findings are confirmed by studies in developing countries where untreated patients present comparable long-term remission rates [8,49]. Long-term seizure remission is less frequent, but still possible, both in men and in women with symptomatic epilepsy (i.e., with seizures associated with a known epileptogenic condition).

Mortality from epilepsy has been found significantly higher in men than in women [50]. In the white population of the USA, the 30-year cumulative standardized mortality ratio was 2.1 (95% CI 1.5–2.8) in men and 1.6 (95% CI 1.1–2.2) in women [51]. Similar observations have been made in developing countries [52], although the data are sparse and flawed. Although the difference can be explained by the differing mortality of the underlying epileptogenic conditions among men and women, further studies are needed to address the reasons for the gender difference in mortality.

Use of antiepileptic drugs

There are only a few studies assessing the use of antiepileptic drugs (AEDs) in the two sexes separately. No major differences have been found between men and women in the total use of AEDs in epilepsy [53–55]. Lamotrigine, gabapentin, and topiramate are used to a greater extent in female than in male patients [53,56], while carbamazepine, valproate, phenytoin, and oxcarbazepine are mostly used in male patients, especially in combination [41,53,57]. No gender differences have been reported for levetiracetam, phenobarbital, and clonazepam [53]. The different tolerability profile (with special reference to weight gain, cosmetic effects, and teratogenicity) may explain the differential use of some AEDs in men and women.

Implications for management

Gender differences do not seem to play a major role in explaining incidence, prevalence, risk factors, and prognosis of epilepsy. Where present, differences between men and women can be found among patients with selected comorbidities (e.g., mood disorders, migraine, multiple sclerosis) and reflect differences in the attributable risk (i.e., the differing number of men and women with a given clinical condition *and* epilepsy reflect the differing distribution of the underlying disease in the two sexes). Although prevention of clinical conditions like stroke, head trauma and infection may affect the risk of seizures and epilepsy, this is unlikely to have a different impact in men and women.

Review of the case: Epidemiological studies provide evidence-based support to the causal association between epilepsy and multiple sclerosis rather than head trauma. Multiple sclerosis carries a threefold risk of seizures while a severe traumatic brain injury that occurred more than 20 years before is unlikely to be a risk factor. Even in patients with symptomatic epilepsy, long-term remission is not unlikely and treatment may be discontinued.

 Key summary points

- The risk of seizures and epilepsy in women is only slightly lower than that of men.
- This slight (nonsignificant) difference may be attributed to the differing distribution of risk factors for epilepsy in men and women and to sociocultural attitudes.
- Some epilepsy syndromes prevail in women and others in men, but the differences tend to disappear in well-defined populations.
- Although the prognosis of epilepsy is similar in the two sexes, the higher mortality of the disease in men may reflect the higher severity of the underlying epileptogenic conditions in the male sex.
- With the aging of the world population and the older average age of women compared to men, an increasing number of women will experience seizures and epilepsy in the future.

References

1 Commission on Epidemiology and Prognosis, International League Against Epilepsy. Guidelines for epidemiologic studies on epilepsy. *Epilepsia* 1993;34:592–596.
2 Fisher RS, van Emde Boas W, Blume W *et al*. Epileptic seizures and epilepsy: definitions proposed by the International League Against Epilepsy (ILAE) and the International Bureau for Epilepsy (IBE). *Epilepsia* 2005;46:470–472.
3 Forsgren L, Beghi E, Oun A, Sillanpaa M. The epidemiology of epilepsy in Europe: a systematic review. *Eur J Neurol* 2005;12:245–253.

4 Sander JW, Hart YM, Johnson AL, Shorvon SD. National General Practice Study of Epilepsy: newly diagnosed epileptic seizures in a general population. *Lancet* 1990;336:1267–1271.

5 Lesser RP. Psychogenic seizures. *Neurology* 1996:46:1499–1507.

6 Preux P-M, Druet-Cabanac M. Epidemiology and etiology of epilepsy in sub-Saharan Africa. *Lancet Neurol* 2005;4:21–31.

7 Cockerell OC, Eckle I, Goodridge DM, Sander JW, Shorvon SD. Epilepsy in a population of 6000 reexamined: secular trends in first attendance rates, prevalence, and prognosis. *J Neurol Neurosurg Psychiatry* 1995;58:570–576.

8 Placencia M, Shorvon SD, Paredes V *et al.* Epileptic seizures in an Andean region of Ecuador. Incidence and prevalence and regional variation. *Brain* 1992;115:771–782.

9 Rwiza HT, Kilonzo GP, Haule J *et al.* Prevalence and incidence of epilepsy in Ulanga, a rural Tanzanian district: a community-based study. *Epilepsia* 1992;33:1051–1056.

10 Sillanpää M, Lastunen S, Helenius H, Schmidt D. Regional differences and secular trends in the incidence of epilepsy in Finland: a nationwide 23-year registry study. *Epilepsia* 2011;52:1857–1867.

11 Hesdorffer DC, Logroscino G, Benn EK, Katri N, Cascino G, Hauser WA. Estimating risk for developing epilepsy: a population-based study in Rochester, Minnesota. *Neurology* 2011;76:23–27.

12 Olafsson E, Ludvigsson P, Gudmundsson G, Hesdorffer D, Kjartansson O, Hauser WA. Incidence of unprovoked seizures and epilepsy in Iceland and assessment of the epilepsy syndrome classification: a prospective study. *Lancet Neurol* 2005;4:627–634.

13 Cowan LD. The epidemiology of the epilepsies in children. *Ment Retard Dev Disabil Res Rev* 2002;8:171–181.

14 Sidenvall R, Forsgren L, Heijbel J. Prevalence and characteristics of epilepsy in children in Northern Sweden. *Seizure* 1996;5:139–146.

15 Granieri E, Rosati G, Tola R *et al.* A descriptive study of epilepsy in the district of Copparo, Italy, 1964–1978. *Epilepsia* 1983;24:502–514.

16 Keränen T, Riekkinen PJ, Sillanpää M. Incidence and prevalence of epilepsy in adults in eastern Finland. *Epilepsia* 1989;30:413–421.

17 Bielen I, Cvitanovic-Sojat L, Bergman-Markovic B *et al.* Prevalence of epilepsy in Croatia: a population-based survey. *Acta Neurol Scand* 2007;116:361–367.

18 Guekht A, Hauser WA, Milchakova L, Churillin Y, Shpak A, Gusev E. The epidemiology of epilepsy in the Russian Federation. *Epilepsy Res* 2010;92:209–218.

19 Panayiotopoulos CP, Obeid T, Tahan AR. Juvenile myoclonic epilepsy: a 5-year prospective study. *Epilepsia* 1994;35:285–296.

20 Zarrelli MM, Beghi E, Rocca WA, Hauser WA. Incidence of epileptic syndromes in Rochester, Minnesota: 1980–1984. *Epilepsia* 1999;40:1708–1714.

21 Josipovic-Jelic Z, Sonicki Z, Soljan I, Demarin V and Collaborative Group for Study of Epilepsy Epidemiology in Sibenik-Knin County, Croatia. Prevalence and socioeconomic aspects of epilepsy in the Croatian county of Sibenik-Knin: community-based survey. *Epilepsy Behav* 2011;20:686–690.

22 Bradford-Hill A. The environment and disease: association or causation? *Proc R Soc Med* 1965;58:295–300.

23 Hauser WA, Hesdorffer DC. Risk factors. In: Hauser WA, Hesdorffer DC (eds) *Epilepsy: Frequency, Causes and Consequences*. New York: Demos Publications, 1990: 53–92.

24 Annegers JF, Hauser WA, Coan SP, Rocca WA. A population-based study of seizures after traumatic brain injuries. *N Engl J Med* 1998;338:20–24.

25 Ounsted C, Lindsay J. The long-term outcome of temporal lobe epilepsy in childhood. In: Reynolds EH, Trimble MR (eds) *Epilepsy and Psychiatry*. Edinburgh: Churchill-Livingstone, 1981: 185–215.

26 Rutter M, Caspi A, Fergusson D *et al*. Sex differences in developmental reading disability: new findings from 4 epidemiological studies. *JAMA* 2004;291:2007–2012.

27 Beghi M, Cornaggia CM, Frigeni B, Beghi E. Learning disorders in epilepsy. *Epilepsia* 2006;47(Suppl 2):14–18.

28 Haut SR, Bigal ME, Lipton RB. Chronic disorders with episodic manifestations: focus on epilepsy and migraine. *Lancet Neurol* 2006;5:148–157.

29 Kaufmann R, Goldberg-Stern H, Shuper A. Attention-deficit disorders and epilepsy in childhood: incidence, causative relations and treatment possibilities. *J Child Neurol* 2009;24:727–733.

30 Gaitatzis A, Trimble MR, Sander JW. The psychiatric comorbidity of epilepsy. *Acta Neurol Scand* 2004;110:207–220.

31 Tellez-Zenteno JF, Patten SB, Jetté N, Williams J, Wiebe S. Psychiatric comorbidity in epilepsy: a population-based analysis. *Epilepsia* 2007;48:2336–2344.

32 Alfstad KÅ, Clench-Aas J, Van Roy B, Mowinckel P, Gjerstad L, Lossius MI. Gender differences in risk-taking behaviour in youth with epilepsy: a Norwegian population-based study. *Acta Neurol Scand Suppl* 2011;191:12–17.

33 Alfstad KÅ, Clench-Aas J, Van Roy B, Mowinckel P, Gjerstad L, Lossius MI. Psychiatric symptoms in Norwegian children with epilepsy aged 8–13 years: effects of age and gender? *Epilepsia* 201;52:1231–1238.

34 Turky A, Beavis JM, Thapar AK, Kerr MP. Psychopathology in children and adolescents with epilepsy: an investigation of predictive variables. *Epilepsy Behav* 2008;12:136–144.

35 Austin JK, Huster G, Dunn DW, Risinger M. Adolescents with active or inactive epilepsy or asthma: a comparison of quality of life. *Epilepsia* 1996;37:1228–1238.

36 McDermott S, Mani S, Krishnaswami S. A population-based analysis of specific behavior problems associated with childhood seizures. *J Epilepsy* 1995;8:110–118.

37 Ettinger AB, Weisbrot DM, Nolan EE *et al*. Symptoms of depression and anxiety in pediatric epilepsy patients. *Epilepsia* 1998;39:595–599.

38 Williams J, Steel C, Sharp GB *et al*. Parental anxiety and quality of life in children with epilepsy. *Epilepsy Behav* 2003;4:729–732.

39 Keene D, Manion I, Whiting S *et al*. A survey of behavior problems in children with epilepsy. *Epilepsy Behav* 2005;6:581–586.

40 Baki O, Erdogan A, Kantarci O, Akisik G, Kayaalp L, Yalcinkaya C. Anxiety and depression in children with epilepsy and their mothers. *Epilepsy Behav* 2004;5:958–964.

41 Gopinath M, Sarma PS, Thomas SV. Gender-specific psychosocial outcome for women with epilepsy. *Epilepsy Behav* 2011;20:44–47.

42 Elwes RD, Marshall J, Beattie A, Newman PK. Epilepsy and employment. A community based survey in an area of high unemployment. *J Neurol Neurosurg Psychiatry* 1991;54:200–203.

43 Marinas A, Elices E, Gil-Nagel A *et al*. Socio-occupational and employment profile of patients with epilepsy. *Epilepsy Behav* 2011;21:223–227.

44 Kim MK, Kwon OY, Cho YW *et al*. Marital status of people with epilepsy in Korea. *Seizure* 2010;19:573–579.

45 Wada K, Iwasa H, Okada M *et al*. Marital status of patients with epilepsy with special reference to the influence of epileptic seizures on the patient's married life. *Epilepsia* 2004;45(Suppl 8):33–36.

46 Jacoby A. Impact of epilepsy on employment status: findings from a UK study of people with well-controlled epilepsy. *Epilepsy Res* 1995;21:125–132.

47 Annegers JF, Hauser WA, Elveback LR. Remission of seizures and relapse in patients with epilepsy. *Epilepsia* 1979;20:729–737.

48 Sillanpää M, Schmidt D. Early seizure frequency and aetiology predict long-term medical outcome in childhood-onset epilepsy. *Brain* 2009;132:989–998.

49 Watts AE. The natural history of untreated epilepsy in a rural community in Africa. *Epilepsia* 1992;33:464–468.

50 Forsgren L, Hauser WA, Olafsson E *et al*. Mortality of epilepsy in developed countries: a review. *Epilepsia* 2005;46(Suppl 1):18–27.

51 Hauser WA, Annegers JF, Elveback LE. Mortality in patients with epilepsy. *Epilepsia* 1980;21:399–412.

52 Carpio A, Barucha NE, Jallon P *et al*. Mortality of epilepsy in developing countries. *Epilepsia* 2005;46(Suppl 1):28–32.

53 Johannessen-Landmark CJ, Fossmark H, Larsson PG, Rytter E, Johannessen SI. Prescription patterns of antiepileptic drugs in patients with epilepsy in a nation-wide population. *Epilepsy Res* 2011;95:51–59.

54 Tsiropoulos B, Gichangi A, Andersen M, Bjerrum L, Gaist D, Hallas J. Trends in utilization of antiepileptic drugs in Denmark. *Acta Neurol Scand* 2006;113:405–411.

55 van de Vrie-Hoekstra NW, de Vries TW, van den Berg PB, Brouwer OF, de Jong-van den Berg LT. Antiepileptic drug utilization in children from 1997 to 2005 a study from the Netherlands. *Eur J Clin Pharmacol* 2008;64:1013–1020.

56 Mattsson P, Tomson T, Eriksson O, Brännström L, Weitoft GR. Sociodemographic differences in antiepileptic drug prescriptions to adult epilepsy patients. *Neurology* 2010;74:295–301.

57 Hollingworth SA, Eadie MJ. Antiepileptic drugs in Australia: 2002–2007. *Pharmacoepidemiol Drug Saf* 2010;19:82–89.

CHAPTER 2

The Social and Psychological Impacts of Epilepsy

Sanjeev V. Thomas[1] and Aparna Nair[2]

[1] Department of Neurology, Sree Chitra Tirunal Institute for Medical Sciences and Technology, Trivandrum, Kerala, India

[2] Centre for Development Studies, Trivandrum, Kerala, India

> **Case History:** *C, a 43-year-old female, was diagnosed with epilepsy when she was 12 years old. Her seizures were controlled with antiepileptic drugs (AEDs). As an adolescent, she did not have many friends and kept mostly to herself. Her teachers described her as withdrawn and isolated, despite being obviously intelligent. Her interactions with her peers became more strained and limited after they witnessed one of her seizures. After finishing school, she opted not to go to university, telling her parents and friends that she did not feel she could manage the challenge well. She took up a low-skilled job that did not pay much but she was able to remain financially independent. By her late twenties she was diagnosed with depression, and also had low self-esteem. In her often short-lived intimate relationships, she was often distant and unable to bond emotionally with her partner. She went on to become increasingly isolated.*

Illness is not merely a physiological state; its impact extends well beyond the physical, biological and medical into the economic, psychological, and social domains of life. It feeds into disease management and overall health status through complex and multidirectional paths. Epilepsy is a typical example of this overlap between the biomedical and psychosocial domains of a disease. The psychosocial impacts of epilepsy have been recognized from the very earliest times, as people with epilepsy have been marginalized in most societies. Nevertheless, there have been many success stories where people have demonstrated extraordinary talents, leadership, and spiritual attainments. Most people with epilepsy are able to enjoy life within their broad community environment. Psychological factors such as stressors, depression, personality traits, and coping mechanisms can impinge on the processes, management and subsequent outcomes of chronic diseases including epilepsy [1,2]. Social consequences of illness (stigma, lower educational attainments and under-employment) can in

Epilepsy in Women, First Edition. Edited by Cynthia L. Harden, Sanjeev V. Thomas and Torbjörn Tomson.

© 2013 John Wiley & Sons, Ltd. Published 2013 by John Wiley & Sons, Ltd.

turn influence access to and utilization of healthcare, as well as increase anxiety and depression [3–6]. An understanding of these non-biomedical impacts is essential for all healthcare professionals who manage epilepsy.

Given that gender has a profound influence on health, illness and healthcare, it is reasonable to hypothesize that females with chronic illnesses would be more vulnerable to these burdens compared with males [7]. Historically, women with epilepsy have experienced the brunt of social and institutional stigmatization and discrimination. In the past there was legislation on marriage, adoption, immigration and the enforced institutionalization of people with epilepsy [8]. Women were the focus of much of this eugenic legislation when epilepsy was legally deemed a "disqualification" for procreation [9]. Disabilities like epilepsy are used to deny citizen's rights to women [10].

In this chapter, we use a life-course perspective to consider how gender influences the social and psychological impacts of living with epilepsy. As women with epilepsy progress through different chronological stages of their lives, the challenges confronted by them and the social, economic, psychological, and familial resources available to them vary. Milestones and transitional events like menarche, puberty, pregnancy and menopause are periods when they are likely to be generally more susceptible to additional stressors, making a life course perspective valuable to the practitioner.

Determinants of the social and psychological impacts of epilepsy

We briefly list some of the physical, medical, social, and cultural factors that are important determinants of the psychosocial impacts of epilepsy in Figure 2.1 and Table 2.1. One important biomedical variable is the level of seizure control: individuals with well-controlled seizures demonstrate lower levels of distress and higher psychosocial functioning and adjustment than those with intractable epilepsy [11]. In addition, variables such as seizure type, type of medication, AED polytherapy, seizure frequency and recency, age of onset, and duration of epilepsy have been linked to the nature of psychosocial adjustment.

The ubiquitous and often powerful stigma associated with epilepsy can have physical consequences, such as increased stress, anxiety and depression. This can additionally influence access to healthcare and/or adherence to medical treatment regimens. Women have been found less likely to seek tertiary medical care for epilepsy within sociocultural contexts where the condition is deeply stigmatizing. The sex ratio (number of women per 1000 men) for people seeking epilepsy care in a tertiary center in South India was 529 while it was 1125 in rural health centers in the same region.

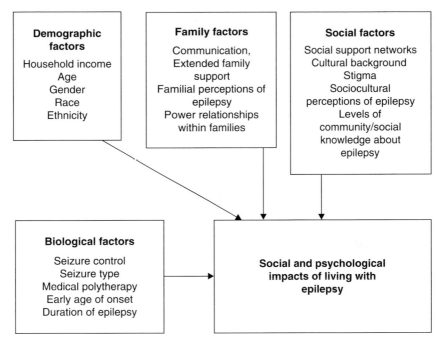

Figure 2.1 Social and psychological impacts of living with epilepsy and its determinants.

This contrast was even more striking among the elderly [12]. The effects of epilepsy-related stigma are mitigated through individual traits such as available access to physical, social, financial, emotional, institutional, and psychological resources. Gender in turn influences how these resources are employed as coping mechanisms. For example, women may find it easier to seek emotional support from their social network, but they may not possess comparable ease of access to financial or institutional resources as male counterparts. In the highly patriarchal South Asian society of Pakistan, research found females with epilepsy less likely to be depressed than males with epilepsy, after considering socioeconomic and marital status, but it is less likely that they possessed autonomy over access to or choice of healthcare [13].

Culture is therefore very relevant to developing a comprehensive understanding of the social and psychological implications of epilepsy for individual patients. Religion, country of origin, ethnicity, group identity, and acculturation are important variables that healthcare professionals should take into consideration. Perceptions of epilepsy are culturally variable, and negative perceptions have been linked to social exclusion and discrimination in addition to influencing care-seeking behavior [14–16]. Cultural affiliations within social groups (such as ethnicity) have been identified as important factors in determining self-efficacy and depression among people with epilepsy [17].

Table 2.1 Social impacts of epilepsy.

Education
Choosing educational trajectory that is not first choice
Disruption of attendance
Inability or impaired ability to reach desired academic goals
Lower educational attainments
Academic under-achievement

Employment
Being in employment that is not first choice
Difficulties in reaching desired career goals
Lower relative employment rates
Difficulties in finding and maintaining employment
Increased absenteeism relative to general population
Lower income
Limitations in/failure to develop ability to live independently

Activity and mobility
Driving
Traveling
Effects of restricted mobility on other domains
Impaired independence
Restricted life

Social interactions and relationships
Failures/difficulties in peer and intimate relationships
Associated stigma among family members
Social withdrawal
Neglect
Social isolation
Discrimination
Exclusion

Psychological
Guilt
Grief
Fear
Anger
Anxiety
Depression
Low self-esteem
Body image
Self-image
Self-concept and identity
Influences psychological development through the life course

Gender itself is socially and culturally contingent, and the roles, expectations and identities allotted to females and males in different sociocultural contexts can influence their health behaviors as well as the way they perceive, understand and treat their epilepsy. In sub-Saharan

Africa, the effects of epilepsy on women's ability to perform socially and economically constructed roles within the community (such as fetching water and cooking on an open fire) contributed to diminished social status [18]. Additionally, culture and gender may influence risk-taking behaviors [19]. In sub-Saharan Africa Baskind and Birbeck [18] observed that the social exclusion of women with epilepsy from the protection afforded by marital relationships pushed them to the outer limits of society, where they were at greater risk of economic and sexual exploitation, and HIV infection. Similar studies from other parts of the world are lacking.

Epilepsy in the female child

The physical manifestations of seizures, the need for continuous use of medications, and its adverse effects as well as the social contexts and meanings of the illness all contribute significantly to the psychosocial burden for young children with epilepsy. At home and in school, children with epilepsy generally fare worse than other children [20]. Social problems are apparent in children with epilepsy: they are less cooperative, less assertive, more withdrawn, and poorer in self-control than healthy children [21]. Gibson [22] pointed out that one of the most important social impacts of childhood epilepsy is the over-protectiveness of parents. This in turn has considerable negative effects on the female child's developing relationship with parents and siblings and on their perceptions of self, as well as their psychological status. In fact, much of the adaptation to epilepsy at this developmental stage depends on the initial reactions of "mediators" (the family, caregivers and healthcare professionals) to the disability [23]. Children with epilepsy demonstrate more behavioral disturbances than children with comparable chronic illnesses including asthma or diabetes [24]. The degree of control achieved over the epilepsy was an important determinant of psychological impacts: children with less controlled epilepsy tend to have poorer self-image, more depression, lower competence, less compliance, and more irritability [23,25].

In school, children with epilepsy often have to deal with the shame over unintended disclosure, bullying, and negative reactions of school staff and peers. This may contribute to academic under-performance [26]. Epilepsy can have a disruptive effect on attendance and performance in academic and extracurricular activities, increasing the potential for social and psychological distress. Educational difficulties may have a longer-term influence on the lives of patients with epilepsy [27].

There is a gender difference in the psychological and social impacts of epilepsy among children. Female children with epilepsy appear to be less susceptible to externalizing behaviors (including behavioral problems at home and in the school) than male children with epilepsy [20]. This may be explained by the finding that psychological problems (particularly depression) show few sex differences; if anything, male children display a higher prevalence of these disorders than female peers [28]. Even the relationship of childhood chronic illness to poor educational attainments and higher risks of unemployment is more pronounced for males than females [27].

The adolescent female with epilepsy

A disability like epilepsy can influence the already turbulent and challenging developmental stage of adolescence in many ways, including the development of psychological problems such as infantilization, the adoption of a sick role, and impaired cognitive function and information processing. Adolescents are also particularly sensitive to stigma; resultant social and psychological problems are more likely during adolescence than childhood [29].

One of the most important social impacts of epilepsy on female adolescents is social isolation [22]. Adolescents with "invisible" disabilities such as epilepsy have difficulties in accepting and sharing their health experiences and are more likely to conceal their epilepsy. This has the potential to influence social relationships, particularly with peers. The propensity to conceal epilepsy continues throughout the life course as a stigma management technique. During adolescence such behavior can contribute to increased psychological and social distress. Unintended disclosure through unexpected, publicly witnessed seizures can further exacerbate the social and psychological impacts of their disability, such as social isolation and withdrawal from peer group activities [30]. However, unintended disclosure through witnessed seizures may well force adolescents with epilepsy to seek out biosocial support groups [22].

Young females with chronic illnesses are more likely to have emotional problems than their healthier counterparts [31]. Adolescent females with epilepsy have more problems with identity, self-image, body image, and ego development than their peers, effects that are exacerbated by disease severity. They tend to internalize symptoms and experience low self-esteem [32]. The unpredictability and intrusiveness of seizures in adolescents translates into periods of intense emotional distress, worry, fear, sadness, anger, and depression [33]. Despite the dual challenges of dealing with adolescence and epilepsy, studies among American adolescents indicated that gender need not necessarily affect self-esteem among young people with epilepsy [34].

In general, the negative psychological and social impacts can be mitigated when adolescents accept epilepsy (or illness/disability) as a natural aspect of life and personal growth that requires ample familial and social support [34]. Therefore, social interactions with important others (doctors, family members, friends, biosocial support groups) are critical in shaping the experience of being diagnosed and the psychological/social implications of living with epilepsy [22]. The physician's role as "mediator" of stigma is particularly vital during adolescence: communication with the adolescent female with epilepsy and her parents is critical in diminishing the effects of perceived and actual stigma [35].

The adult female with epilepsy

Adulthood presents women with another set of experiences, challenges and concerns. This developmental stage in women's lives involves the challenges of developing personal/professional identities, finishing advanced education, finding suitable employment, establishing relationships with partners, having children, and finding a foothold in their careers, in addition to managing their epilepsy. The transition to adulthood may involve separation from the natal family unit and a greater dependence on the self for all aspects of epilepsy management. This can result in biological, psychological and social consequences, including loneliness, enforced social isolation, anxiety, and worry [22].

On the economic front, gender may influence everything from educational attainments to the acquisition of marketable skills, employment and wages [36]. In the USA, epilepsy is an important employment deterrent for adult females and males but more profoundly for males. However, the situation becomes more complex for adult females in the workforce when they must manage the demands of partnerships and child-rearing [37].

Research suggests that success or failure in education, employment and social status may predict the psychological and social consequences of epilepsy in adulthood. Women with epilepsy of childbearing age are at higher risk of depression compared to women without epilepsy, particularly if they are unemployed or have had seizures in the near past, but are not at higher risk for depression compared to males with epilepsy [38]. The latter finding is surprising given the commonly replicated research finding that women in the reproductive age group are roughly twice as vulnerable to clinically significant depression as males of the same ages [28,39,40].

Gender tends to influence the social indicators such as marital status among adult women with epilepsy, but studies have been inconclusive. While one study found that males with epilepsy were less likely to be married than females with epilepsy, another study found no significant gender differences in the likelihood of being married [41]. Cultural background can influence the relationship between gender, epilepsy, and intimate relationships including marriage. Epilepsy can strain the relationship between partners if the woman with epilepsy is unable to fulfil her socioculturally determined and individually varying roles as partner and/or mother. Adult females with epilepsy are also arguably more vulnerable to adverse social and psychological effects when they confront difficulties in conceiving and rearing children as a result of their illness.

The middle-aged group is considered a "sandwich" generation: the developmental tasks at this stage include providing emotional and financial support to partners and/or children, mentoring relationships with the next generation in the workplace, accepting and adjusting to physiological changes, and providing emotional support to and sometimes caring for aging parents. Older adults may have more difficulty coping with epilepsy than younger patients, who have more physiological reserves and fewer responsibilities; older patients may also have to cope with decrements in health status because of other comorbid illnesses [42,43]. Further, the fluctuations in female hormones that accompany menopause have been linked to worsening of seizures in some women [44]. First-person narratives of epilepsy suggest that as middle-aged women approach menopause, their apprehensions about the effects of this major biological change on their epilepsy could also result in anxiety, worry and depression [45].

The elderly female with epilepsy

The incidence of epilepsy is highest among the elderly [46]. Older females tend to have more negative affect, which in turn could result in lower perceived quality of life when illness is chronic [47]. The elderly woman with epilepsy must confront other psychosocial challenges. Social-breakdown theory argues that the aged are more vulnerable to social labeling than at other stages in their life, which in turn results in increasingly negative perceptions of the self. Subsequently, relatively trivial events can snowball into serious, life-altering problems for older adults [48]. Given the higher risks of disease morbidity among older populations in general, the onset of epilepsy in this age group is likely to add to the psychological and social burdens of comorbidities in complex ways. Older females with epilepsy find it more difficult to confront the stigma associated with diagnosis and the physical manifestations of epilepsy than male counterparts [49]. Among newly diagnosed older persons with epilepsy, the very old (>85 years) have lower quality of life than those aged 65–74 years [50]. Social withdrawal and/or isolation at this point in the lives of female patients can prove an additional challenge, as could the loss of confidence and reduced independence resulting from the loss of driving licenses. In countries where assisted living is common, epilepsy can contribute to premature admission of individuals to nursing homes or assisted living facilities [51]. The increasing dependence on their social support networks becomes a matter of concern. Older women with newly diagnosed epilepsy require particular attention to their mental health as they have higher risk of depression than those with long-standing epilepsy.

Review of the case: *The case history presented earlier in this chapter is intended to demonstrate how the psychosocial burden of epilepsy changes as an individual progresses through the life course. In this instance, stigma associated with seizures and unintended behavior/neglect from peers aggravated her social isolation during adolescence, resulting in lifelong psychological consequences. She quit pursuing her education, which in turn had a serious negative impact on her socioeconomic status. She grew up with low self-esteem and failed to establish strong and healthy partnerships. Proper understanding of the illness among her social network and judicious disclosure of her epilepsy eventually contributed to better psychological and social outcomes. She identified and joined a biosocial support group where the interactions with other women who lived successful lives in spite of epilepsy helped her to come out of her self-imposed isolation. She signed up for night classes and began pursuing a college degree in education.*

 Key summary points

- As patients move from childhood to adolescence to adulthood and later, the psychological and social implications of living with epilepsy change.
  - The family plays a crucial role in determining how children with epilepsy perceive and respond to their conditions.
  - Young children with epilepsy are prone to poorer self-image, depression, less compliance, and more irritability than children without epilepsy.
  - As they transition to adolescence, females with epilepsy become more vulnerable to the psychological impacts and social consequences of their disability.
  - The transition to a more independent individual adult can be particularly difficult for young females with epilepsy who rely only on their social network for care.
  - Adult women confront challenges in acquiring educational goals, employment, sustaining intimate relationships, and having children. This age group is particularly at risk of psychological distress if there are perceived failures in the above domains.
  - As women approach menopause, they need to be counseled regarding the increasing claims on their physical, social, economic, and psychological resources that may render them particularly vulnerable to the psychosocial burdens of epilepsy.
  - Elderly women with epilepsy are particularly vulnerable to stigmatization, social exclusion, premature admission into institutions, loss of mobility/independence, and consequent distress.
- Equally critical is a physician's knowledge of the sociocultural backgrounds of patients and their families.
- Physicians should be active in encouraging and facilitating the creation of biosocial support groups within and outside institutional settings, where women with epilepsy are able to share their experiences and concerns with others who have had similar experiences.

References

1 Williams RB, Schneiderman N. Resolved: psychosocial interventions can improve clinical outcomes in organic disease progression. *Psychosom Med* 2002;64:552–557.

2 Leserman J, Petitto JM, Golden RN *et al.* Impact of stressful life events, depression, social support, coping, and cortisol on progression to AIDS. *Am J Psychiatry* 2000;157:1221–1228.

3 Charmaz K. Loss of self: a fundamental form of suffering in the chronically ill. *Sociol Health Illn* 1983;5:168–195.

4 Hermann BP. Quality of life in epilepsy. *J Epilepsy* 1992;5:153–165.

5 Jacoby A, Baker GA, Steen N, Potts P, Chadwick DW. The clinical course of epilepsy and its psychosocial correlates: findings from a UK community study. *Epilepsia* 1996;37:148–161.

6 Baker, GA. The psychosocial burden of epilepsy. *Epilepsia* 2002;43:26–30.

7 Johnson JL, Greaves L, Repta R. Better science with sex and gender: facilitating the use of a sex and gender-based analysis in health research. *Int J Equity Health* 2009;8:1–11.

8 Stirling J. *Representing Epilepsy: Myth and Matter.* Liverpool: Liverpool University Press, 2010.

9 Kline W. *Building a Better Race: Gender, Sexuality and Eugenics from the Turn of the Nineteenth Century to the Baby Boom.* Berkeley: University of California Press, 2001.

10 Baynton DC. Disability and the justification of inequality in American history. In: Longmore P, Umansky L (eds) *The New Disability History: American Perspectives.* New York: New York University Press, 2001: 33–57.

11 Jacoby A. Epilepsy and the quality of everyday life: findings from a study of people with well-controlled epilepsy. *Soc Sci Med* 1992;34:657–668.

12 Thomas SV, Deetha TD, Nair P, Sarma SP. Fewer women receive tertiary care for epilepsy in Kerala state, India. *Epileptic Disord* 2006;8:184–189.

13 Yousafzai AR, Yousafzai AW, Taj R. Frequency of depression in epilepsy: a hospital-based study. *J Ayub Med Coll Abbottabad* 2009;21:73–75.

14 Buck D, Jacoby A, Baker GA, Ley H, Steen N. Cross-cultural differences in health-related quality of life of people with epilepsy: findings from a European study. *Qual Life Res* 1999;8:675–685.

15 Nuhu FT, Fawole JO, Babalola OJ, Ayilara OO, Sulaiman ZT. Social consequences of epilepsy: a study of 231 Nigerian patients. *Ann Afr Med* 2010;9:170–175.

16 Mushi D, Hunter E, Mtuya C, Mshana G, Aris E, Walker R. Social-cultural aspects of epilepsy in Kilimanjaro Region, Tanzania: knowledge and experience among patients and carers. *Epilepsy Behav* 2011;20:338–343.

17 Chong J, Drake K, Atkinson PB, Ouellette E, Labiner DM. Social and family characteristics of Hispanics with epilepsy. *Seizure* 2012;21:12–16.

18 Baskind R, Birbeck GL. Epilepsy-associated stigma in sub-Saharan Africa: the social landscape of a disease. *Epilepsy Behav* 2005;7:68–73.

19 Hahn RA, Teutsch SM, Franks AL, Chang MH, Lloyd EE. The prevalence of risk factors among women in the United States by race and age, 1992–1994: opportunities for primary and secondary prevention. *J Am Med Women's Assoc* 1998;53: 96–104, 107.

20 Carlton-Ford S, Miller R, Brown M, Nealeigh N, Jennings P. Epilepsy and children's social and psychological adjustment. *J Health Soc Behav* 1995;36:285–301.

21 Hamiwka LD, Hamiwka LA, Sherman EM, Wirrell E. Social skills in children with epilepsy: how do they compare to healthy and chronic disease controls? *Epilepsy Behav* 2011;21:238–241.

22 Gibson PA. The impact of epilepsy on relationships. In: Morrell MJ (ed.) *Women with Epilepsy: A Handbook of Health and Treatment Issues*. Cambridge: Cambridge University Press, 2003: 237–249.

23 Austin JK, McBride AB, Davis HW. Parental attitude and adjustment to childhood epilepsy. *Nurs Res* 1984;33:92–96.

24 Austin JK, Smith MS, Risinger MW, McNelis AM. Childhood epilepsy and asthma: comparison of quality of life. *Epilepsia* 1994;35:608–615.

25 Austin JK. Huberty TJ. Development of the child attitude toward illness scale. *J Pediatr Psychol* 1993;18:467–480.

26 Moffat C, Dorris L, Connor L, Espie CA. The impact of childhood epilepsy on quality of life: a qualitative investigation using focus group methods to obtain children's perspectives on living with epilepsy. *Epilepsy Behav* 2009;14:179–189.

27 Pless I, Power C, Peckham C. Long-term psychosocial sequelae of chronic physical disorders in childhood. *Pediatrics* 1993;91:1131–1136.

28 Maughan, B. Depression and psychological distress: a life course approach. In: Kuh D, Hardy R (eds) *A Life Course Approach to Women's Health*. Oxford: Oxford University Press, 2002:161–176.

29 Westbrook LE, Bauman LJ, Shinnar S. Applying stigma theory to epilepsy: a test of a conceptual model. *J Pediatr Psychol* 1992;17:633–649.

30 Pless I, Roghmann K. Chronic illness and its consequences: observations based on three epidemiologic surveys. *J Pediatr* 1971;79:351–359.

31 Surís J, Parera N, Puig C. Chronic illness and emotional distress in adolescence. *J Adolesc Health* 1996;19:153–156.

32 Michaud P-A, Suris JC, Viner R. *The Adolescent with a Chronic Condition: Epidemiology, Developmental Issues and Healthcare Provision*. WHO Discussion Papers on Adolescence. Geneva: World Health Organization, 2007.

33 Elliott I, Lach L, Smith M. I just want to be normal: a qualitative study exploring how children and adolescents view the impact of intractable epilepsy on their quality of life. *Epilepsy Behav* 2005;7:664–678.

34 Berntsson L, Berg M, Brydolf M, Hellstrom AL. Adolescent's experiences of well-being when living with long-term illness or disability. *Scand J Caring Sci* 2007;21:419–425.

35 Baker GA, Jacoby A. The stigma of epilepsy: implications for clinical management. In: Mason T, Carlisle C, Watkins C, Whitehead E (eds) *Stigma and Social Exclusion in Healthcare*. New York: Routledge, 2001:126–136.

36 Famulari M. The effects of a disability on labor market performance: the case of epilepsy. *Southern Econ J* 1992;58:1972–1087.

37 Troxell J. Work issues and epilepsy. In: Morrell MJ (ed.) *Women with Epilepsy: A Handbook of Health and Treatment Issues*. Cambridge: Cambridge University Press, 2003:281–287.

38 Beghi E, Roncolato M, Visonà G. Depression and altered quality of life in women with epilepsy of childbearing age. *Epilepsia* 2004;45:64–70.

39 Grabowska-Grzyb A, Jedrzejczak J, Naganska E, Fiszer U. Risk factors for depression in patients with epilepsy. *Epilepsy Behav* 2006;8:411–417.

40 Thompson AW, Miller JW, Katon W, Chaytor N, Ciechanowski P. Sociodemographic and clinical factors associated with depression in epilepsy. *Epilepsy Behav* 2009;14: 655–660.

41 Elliott JO, Charyton C, McAuley JW, Shneker BF. The impact of marital status on epilepsy-related health concerns. *Epilepsy Res* 2011;95:200–206.

42 Pugh MJV, Copeland LA, Zeyer JE *et al*. The impact of epilepsy on health status among younger and older adults. *Epilepsia* 2005;26:1820–1827.

43 Kingsmill S, Schlesinger B. *The Family Squeeze: Surviving the Sandwich Generation.* Toronto: University of Toronto Press, 1998.

44 Abbasi F, Krumholz A. Menopause and epilepsy. In: Morrell MJ (ed.) *Women with Epilepsy: A Handbook of Health and Treatment Issues.* Cambridge: Cambridge University Press, 2003:131–145.

45 Lindahl LZ. On being a woman with epilepsy. In: Morrell MJ (ed.) *Women with Epilepsy: A Handbook of Health and Treatment Issues.* Cambridge: Cambridge University Press, 2003:7–17.

46 Hauser WA. Seizure disorders: the changes with age. *Epilepsia* 1992;33:6–14.

47 Efklides A, Kalaitzidou M, Chankin G. Subjective quality of life in old age in Greece: the effect of demographic factors, emotional state and adaptation to aging. *Eur Psychol* 2003;8:178–191.

48 Kuypers JA, Bengtson VL. Social breakdown and competence: a model of normal aging. *Hum Dev* 1973;16:181–201.

49 Baker GA, Jacoby A, Buck D, Brooks J, Potts P, Chadwick DW. The quality of life of older people with epilepsy: findings from a UK community study. *Seizure* 2001;10:92–99.

50 Martin R, Vogtle L, Gilliam F, Faught E. Health-related quality of life in senior adults with epilepsy: what we know from randomized clinical trials and suggestions for future research. *Epilepsy Behav* 2003;4:626–634.

51 Brodie MJ. Kwan P. Epilepsy in elderly people. *Br Med J* 2005;331:1317–1322.

CHAPTER 3

Neurosteroid Influences on Neuronal Excitability: The Menstrual Cycle and Catamenial Epilepsy as Dynamic Models

Doodipala Samba Reddy

Department of Neuroscience and Experimental Therapeutics, College of Medicine, Texas A&M Health Science Center, Bryan, Texas, USA

Introduction

Steroid hormones play an important role in neuronal excitability and seizure susceptibility. Neurosteroids are steroids synthesized within the brain with unconventional rapid effects on neuronal excitability. The term *neurosteroid* was coined in 1981 by the French endocrinologist Étienne-Émile Baulieu to refer to steroids that are synthesized *de novo* in the nervous system from cholesterol independent of the peripheral steroidogenic endocrine glands [1]. Subsequently, the term *neuroactive steroid* has been widely used to describe natural or synthetic steroids that rapidly alter the excitability of neurons by binding to membrane-bound receptors. It has been known since the 1940s, from the pioneering work of Hans Selye, that naturally occurring steroids such as the ovarian steroid progesterone and the adrenal steroid deoxycorticosterone (DOC) can exert anesthetic and anticonvulsant actions [2]. In the early 1980s, the synthetic steroid alfaxalone was found to enhance synaptic inhibition via γ-aminobutyric acid (GABA)-A receptors in the brain [3]. A major advance occurred when 5α-reduced metabolites of progesterone and DOC were also found to enhance GABA-A receptor function [4]. It was speculated that the anesthetic and anticonvulsant properties of progesterone and DOC were due to their conversion to allopregnanolone (3α-hydroxy-5α-pregnan-20-one, AP) and allotetrahydrodeoxycorticosterone (3α,21-dihydroxy-5α-pregnan-20-one, THDOC), respectively [5]. The androgenic neurosteroid androstanediol (5α-androstan-3α,17β-diol) is synthesized from testosterone [6].

Epilepsy in Women, First Edition. Edited by Cynthia L. Harden, Sanjeev V. Thomas and Torbjörn Tomson.
© 2013 John Wiley & Sons, Ltd. Published 2013 by John Wiley & Sons, Ltd.

Table 3.1 Summary of steroid hormone modulation of seizure susceptibility.

Hormone	Actions	Potential mechanisms of action
Estrogens	Proconvulsant	Hippocampal dendritic spine density
		Enhanced NMDA receptor function
Progesterone	Anticonvulsant	Neurosteroid AP precursor
		Potentiation of GABA-A receptor function
Androgens	Proconvulsant and	Estrogen precursor (proconvulsant)
	anticonvulsant	Androstanediol precursor (anticonvulsant)
Deoxycorticosterone	Anticonvulsant	Neurosteroid THDOC precursor
		Potentiation of GABA-A receptor function
Cortisol	Proconvulsant	Corticosteroid receptors and plasticity
AP	Anticonvulsant	Potentiation of GABA-A receptor function
THDOC	Anticonvulsant	Potentiation of GABA-A receptor function
Androstanediol	Anticonvulsant	Potentiation of GABA-A receptor function
Pregnenolone sulfate	Proconvulsant	Inhibition of GABA-A receptor function
		Potentiation of NMDA receptor function
DHEA sulfate	Proconvulsant	Inhibition of GABA-A receptor function
		Potentiation of NMDA receptor function

DHEA, dehydroepiandrosterone; NMDA, *N*-methyl-D-aspartate; other abbreviations defined in the text.

There is now compelling evidence that all the enzymes required for the biosynthesis of the neurosteroids from cholesterol are present in the brain. Since neurosteroids are highly lipophilic and can readily cross the blood–brain barrier, neurosteroids synthesized in peripheral tissues accumulate in the brain. Neurosteroids and their precursor steroid hormones play an important role in the neuronal excitability, seizure susceptibility, and pathophysiology of neurological conditions such as catamenial epilepsy (Table 3.1). This chapter describes the menstrual cycle, steroid hormones, and neuroendocrinological aspects of catamenial epilepsy, a menstrual cycle-related seizure disorder in women with epilepsy. A clinical discussion of catamenial epilepsy and current treatment approaches are fully discussed in Chapter 4.

The menstrual cycle

The average menstrual cycle is about 28 days (range 24–35 days). The normal cycle proceeds through various phases based on the neuroendocrine changes. Ovulation normally occurs mid-cycle, around day 14. Using the first day of menstrual bleeding as the first day of the cycle, the menstrual cycle is divided into four phases: (i) menstrual phase, days −3 to +3; (ii) follicular phase, days +4 to +9; (iii) ovulatory phase, days +10 to +16; and (iv) luteal phase, days +17 to −4. Figure 3.1(a) shows the neuroendocrine pathways of estrogen and progesterone production during the menstrual cycle [7].

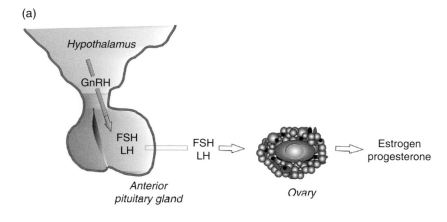

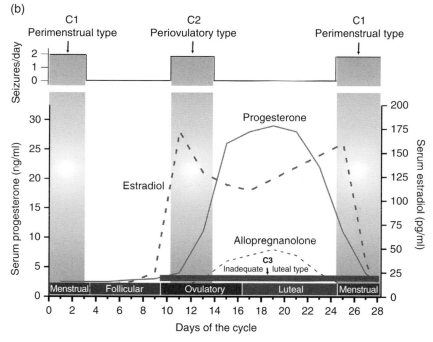

Figure 3.1 Sex hormone levels and seizure susceptibility during the menstrual cycle. (a) Neuroendocrine pathways of steroid hormone production. The synthesis and secretion of estrogens and progesterone from the ovaries is controlled primarily by hypothalamic gonadotropin-releasing hormone (GnRH) and pituitary gonadotropins. GnRH stimulates the synthesis and release of the gonadotropins follicle-stimulating hormone (FSH) and luteinizing hormone (LH) from the anterior pituitary gland in a pulsatile fashion. FSH and LH stimulate the development of ovarian follicles, ovulation, and production of estrogens and progesterone. (b) Temporal relationship between ovarian hormones and occurrence of catamenial seizures. The upper panel illustrates the strong relationship between seizure frequency and estradiol/progesterone levels. The lower panel illustrates the three types of catamenial epilepsy. The vertical gray bars to left and right represent the likely period for the perimenstrual (C1) type, while the vertical gray bar in the middle represents the likely period for the periovulatory (C2) type. The horizontal dark gray bar (bottom) represents the inadequate luteal (C3) type that likely occurs between the early ovulatory and menstrual phases.

During the follicular phase, the primary outcome is development of a follicle capable of achieving ovulation successfully. The follicle-stimulating hormone (FSH) levels are greatly increased to initiate growth of immature ovarian follicles. FSH, luteinizing hormone (LH), and estrogen influence the ovarian follicle to secrete estrogen. Estrogen production inhibits FSH secretion, therefore reducing the amount of FSH toward the end of the follicular phase. The high levels of estrogen cause the endometrium to thicken, which will later lead to the layer shedding if the ovum is not fertilized. As the ovulatory phase begins, LH begins to rise toward its peak. The high levels of estrogen cause a sudden flow of LH secretion that results in ovulation of the mature follicle and an increase in progesterone. Estrogen levels suddenly drop once the follicle reaches the ovulation phase. As the luteal phase approaches, there are high levels of progesterone and moderate levels of estrogen secreted by the corpus luteum. Progesterone inhibits FSH and LH, which are at very low levels during this phase. The corpus luteum degenerates within 2 weeks if the ovum is not fertilized, resulting in a sharp decrease in progesterone and estrogen levels. Since progesterone is no longer inhibiting FSH and LH, the levels of these two anterior pituitary hormones start to increase, starting the cycle again. The menstrual phase is characterized by the demise of the corpus luteum and shedding of the endometrium, when bleeding occurs. The shedding of the endometrial layer is caused by the sudden absence of estrogen and progesterone. Some women may experience anovulatory cycles. Abnormal FSH secretion may lead to inadequate follicular development and thus subnormal functioning of the corpus luteum, a condition referred to as "inadequate luteal-phase," usually associated with anovulation. Progesterone levels are very low in this scenario and could alter the neuroendocrine inhibitory mechanisms.

Catamenial epilepsy

A hallmark of epilepsy is the unpredictable occurrence of seizures. However, in many women with epilepsy, seizures do not occur randomly but cluster in association with the menstrual cycle. This condition is referred to as *catamenial epilepsy*. Catamenial epilepsy is a neuroendocrine condition in which seizures are clustered around specific points in the menstrual cycle, most often the perimenstrual or periovulatory periods. Catamenial epilepsy affects 10–70% of women with epilepsy [7–10]. The large variation in the prevalence of catamenial epilepsy is partly because of methodological differences such as the criteria used for defining seizure exacerbation in relation to the menstrual cycle, patient self-reporting, diaries, and other records of seizures relating to menses. Overall, these studies support the prevailing notion that at least one in every three

Table 3.2 Three patterns of catamenial epilepsy.

C1: perimenstrual
Characterized by a greater average daily seizure frequency during the menstrual phase (day −3 to +3) compared with the mid-follicular (day 4 to 9) and mid-luteal (day −12 to 14) phases in normal ovulatory cycles
Incidence: High

C2: periovulatory
Characterized by a greater average daily seizure frequency during the ovulatory phase (day 10 to −13) compared with the mid-follicular and mid-luteal phases in normal ovulatory cycles
Incidence: Medium

C3: Inadequate luteal-phase
Characterized by a greater seizure frequency during the ovulatory, luteal, and menstrual phases than during the mid-folliclar phase in women with inadequate (anovulatory) luteal-phase cycles
Incidence: Low-Medium

---

women with epilepsy shows catamenial seizure exacerbation. Catamenial epilepsy is a form of intractable epilepsy because catamenial seizures are often quite resistant to available drug treatments. Despite new developments, presently there is no effective prevention or cure for catamenial epilepsy. There is a large gap in our understanding of what changes occur in the brain in relation to the hormonal fluctuations associated with catamenial epilepsy and how these changes alter sensitivity to anticonvulsant drugs. Thus, a detailed understanding of the patterns and pathophysiology is essential for the development of rational approaches for the prevention or treatment of catamenial epilepsy.

Three types of catamenial seizures have been identified: perimenstrual (C1), periovulatory (C2), and inadequate luteal-phase (C3) [11] (Figure 3.1b and Table 3.2). The perimenstrual type is the most common clinical type. Perimenstrual and periovulatory types are illustrated in Figure 3.1(b). The specific pattern of catamenial epilepsy can be identified simply by charting menses and seizures and obtaining a mid-luteal phase serum progesterone level to distinguish between normal and inadequate luteal-phase cycles [12,13]. A designation of catamenial epilepsy can be made if a twofold or greater increase in seizure frequency is observed during a particular phase of the menstrual cycle. In the primary clinical type, perimenstrual catamenial epilepsy, women with epilepsy experience an increase in seizure activity before, during or after the onset of menstruation [7]. Catamenial epilepsy is observed in women with ovulatory or anovulatory cycles. Women with ovulatory cycles could experience the perimenstrual, periovulatory, or even both catamenial types within a single cycle [14,15]. About 16.5% of cycles in study subjects are found to be anovulatory [8], and these women showed a third type, referred to as inadequate luteal-phase or anovulatory luteal seizures. For accurate diagnosis, records of a 3-month period during which patients note seizures and menstrual onset on a calendar are essential. A mid-luteal phase serum progesterone level is obtained within 4–12 days prior to menses. A level below 5 ng/mL is used to designate anovulatory or inadequate luteal-phase cycles.

Neuroendocrine aspects of catamenial epilepsy

Catamenial epilepsy is a multifaceted condition attributed to numerous causes. Epilepsy typically develops due to certain genetic defects or often after a presumed initiating injury. In many cases, catamenial epilepsy is assumed to be an acquired disorder and currently there is no clear evidence of genetic components. A variety of mechanisms, such as fluctuations in antiepileptic drug levels, changes in water and electrolyte balance, and physiological variation in ovarian hormone secretion, have been proposed as causes for catamenial epilepsy [7,16]. Overall, cyclical changes in the circulating levels of estrogens and progesterone are now widely accepted to play a central role in the development of this condition (Figure 3.1). Generally, estrogens are found to be proconvulsant, while progesterone has powerful antiseizure effects and reduces seizures, thus playing a central role in the pathophysiology of catamenial epilepsy. There is emerging evidence that endogenous neurosteroids influence seizure susceptibility in epilepsy [5].

Role of estrogens
The role of estrogens in seizure susceptibility is complex. In general, estrogens have proconvulsant and epileptogenic properties in animals and humans. There are also studies that support protective effects of estrogens and it may also be anticonvulsant under some circumstances. Estradiol has been widely investigated in animal epilepsy models. However, the effect of estrogens on seizure susceptibility is highly variable and depends on factors such as treatment duration, dosage, hormonal status, and the seizure model [17]. Early studies of estradiol administration to ovariectomized rats revealed proconvulsant effects [7]. The effect of estrogens on hippocampus seizure susceptibility is controversial. While estradiol has been shown to be proconvulsant in several studies, there is also evidence that supports a lack of effect or protective effect of estrogens [18,19]. In low doses, estradiol can produce neuroprotective effects [19].

Estradiol has been known to play a role in the exacerbation of seizures in women with epilepsy [13,20–23]. Plasma estradiol levels are found to increase during both the follicular and luteal phase of the normal menstrual cycle (Figure 3.1). Bäckström [21] was the first investigator to characterize the relationship between seizures and steroid hormones. In women with epilepsy, a positive correlation between seizure susceptibility and the ratio of estrogen to progesterone was observed, peaking in the premenstrual and preovulatory periods and declining during the mid-luteal phase. Logothetis *et al.* [20] have demonstrated that intravenous infusions of estrogen are associated with rapid interictal epileptiform activity in women with epilepsy and that seizures are exacerbated when estrogen is given premenstrually. Therefore, it is hypothesized that estrogens may facilitate some forms of catamenial seizures observed during these phases. The periovulatory catamenial exacerbation has been attributed to the mid-cycle surge of estrogen that is relatively unopposed by progesterone until the early luteal phase [20]. An increase in the ratio of estrogen to progesterone levels during the perimenstrual period (described below) might at least partly contribute to the development of perimenstrual seizure exacerbation [11,22]. Nevertheless, the exact relationship between circulating estrogens and perimenstrual or anovulatory catamenial seizures remains unclear.

Role of progesterone

Progesterone (P) plays a key role in catamenial epilepsy. Progesterone has consistent anticonvulsant and antiepileptic properties in animals and humans. Progesterone has long been known to have antiseizure activity in a variety of animal models of epilepsy [24,25]. In recent years, numerous studies have confirmed the powerful anticonvulsant activity of progesterone in diverse animal seizure models [7]. There is strong evidence that the antiseizure effects of progesterone are not related to interactions with classical progesterone receptors (PRs), because the antiseizure activity of progesterone is undiminished in PR knockout mice [26]. Further studies established that 5α-reduced metabolites of progesterone, particularly AP, are responsible for the seizure protection conferred by progesterone. Recent studies in our laboratory confirm the antiepileptogenic effects of progesterone in the kindling model of epileptogenesis [27]. Consequently, seizure susceptibility is very low during physiological conditions associated with high progesterone.

In women with epilepsy, natural cyclic variations in progesterone during the menstrual cycle could influence catamenial seizure susceptibility (Figure 3.1). Seizures decrease in the mid-luteal phase when serum progesterone levels are high and increase premenstrually when progesterone levels fall and there is a decrease in the serum progesterone-to-estrogen ratio [12,22,23]. Changes in progesterone levels have been directly correlated with catamenial seizures [28,29]. Despite some limitations, these findings provide evidence that disruption in ovarian cycle-related fluctuations in progesterone can be correlated to catamenial seizure exacerbation. The emerging evidence clearly indicates that perimenstrual catamenial seizures are associated with a rapid decline in progesterone around menstruation.

Role of neurosteroids

Progesterone is a precursor for the synthesis of neurosteroids in the brain. Neurosteroids are steroids that rapidly alter neuronal excitability through nongenomic mechanisms. Recent work has demonstrated that the anti-convulsant properties of progesterone and adrenal DOC are due to their conversion to the neurosteroids AP and THDOC, respectively [5]. A variety of neurosteroids are known to be synthesized in the brain. The most widely studied are AP, THDOC, and androstanediol. They are produced via sequential A-ring reduction of steroid hormones by 5α-reductase and 3α-hydroxysteroid oxidoreductase isoenzymes. In the periphery, the steroid precursors are mainly synthesized in the gonads, adrenal gland, and fetoplacental unit, but synthesis of these neurosteroids likely occurs in the brain from cholesterol or from peripherally derived intermediates. Since neurosteroids are highly lipophilic and can readily cross the blood–brain barrier, neurosteroids synthesized in peripheral tissues accumulate in the brain.

Recent evidence indicates that neurosteroids are present mainly in principal neurons in many brain regions that are relevant to focal epilepsies, including the hippocampus and neocortex [30,31]. The highly restricted distribution of neurosteroids to excitatory neurons suggests that they are mainly derived from local synthesis, although it is clear that peripheral neurosteroids easily cross the blood–brain barrier. The biosynthesis of neuro-steroids is controlled by the translocator protein (18kDa; TSPO), formerly called the peripheral or mitochondrial benzodiazepine receptor [32]. Activation of TSPO by endogenous signals and ligands facilitates the intrami-tochondrial flux of cholesterol and thereby promotes neurosteroid synthesis. Neurosteroids are localized to the neurons that contain their target receptors, which is consistent with the concept that neurosteroids function in an auto-crine fashion in which they reach their targets by lateral membrane diffusion.

Neurosteroid interaction with synaptic and extrasynaptic GABA-A receptors is illustrated in Figure 3.2. Neurosteroids rapidly alter neuronal excitability through direct interaction with GABA-A receptors [33–35], which are the major receptors for the inhibitory neurotransmitter GABA. Activation of the GABA-A receptor by various ligands leads to an influx of chloride (Cl⁻) ions and to hyperpolarization of the membrane that dampens the excitability. AP and other structurally related neurosteroids act as positive allosteric modulators and direct activators of GABA-A receptors. At low concentrations, neurosteroids potentiate GABA-A receptor currents, whereas at higher concentrations they directly activate the receptor [36,37]. Like barbiturates, neurosteroid enhancement of GABA-A

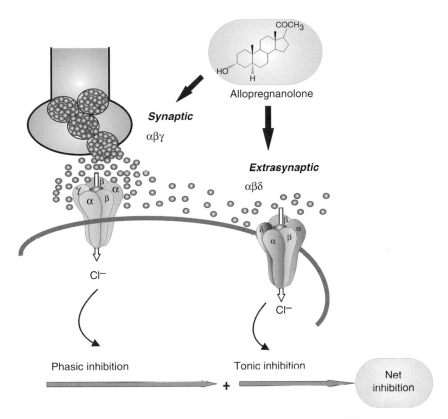

Figure 3.2 Neurosteroid modulation of synaptic and extrasynaptic GABA-A receptors. Postsynaptic GABA-A receptors, which are pentameric chloride channels composed of 2α2βγ subunits, mediate the phasic portion of GABAergic inhibition, while extrasynaptic GABA-A receptors, pentamers composed of 2α2βδ subunits, primarily contribute to tonic inhibition in the hippocampus. Neurosteroids, such as AP, binds to the "neurosteroid binding sites", which are distinct from sites for GABA, benzodiazepines, and barbiturates. Neurosteroids activate both synaptic and extrasynaptic receptors and enhance the phasic and tonic inhibition, and thereby promote maximal net inhibition. Such potentiation of the GABAergic inhibition underlies neurosteroid protective actions against epileptic seizures.

receptors occurs through increases in both the channel open frequency and channel open duration.

The GABA-A receptor is a pentamer consisting of five subunits that form a chloride channel. Sixteen subunits (α1–6, β1–3, γ1–3, δ, ε, θ, and π subunits) have been identified so far. The GABA site is located at the interface between the α and β subunits. Benzodiazepines bind at the interface between the α and γ subunits and they interact with subunit combinations α1,2,3, or 5+β2+γ2. The effect of neurosteroids on GABA-A receptors occurs by binding to discrete sites on the receptor–channel complex that are located within the transmembrane domains of the α and β subunits [33,34], which they access by lateral membrane diffusion [38,39]. The binding sites for neurosteroids are distinct from the recognition sites for GABA, benzodiazepines, and barbiturates [6,35]. The GABA-A receptor mediates two types of GABAergic inhibition, now stratified into synaptic (phasic) or extrasynaptic (tonic) inhibition (Figure 3.2). Although GABA activates synaptic (γ2-containing) GABA-A receptors with high efficacy, GABA activation of the extrasynaptic (δ-containing) GABA-A receptors is limited to low-efficacy activity, characterized by minimal desensitization and brief openings. Although neurosteroids act on all GABA-A receptor isoforms, they have large effects on extrasynaptic δ-subunit-containing GABA-A receptors that mediate tonic currents [40,41]. Consequently, GABA-A receptors that contain the δ-subunit are highly sensitive to neurosteroid potentiation. Tonic currents cause a steady inhibition of neurons and reduce their excitability. Therefore, neurosteroids could play a role in setting the level of excitability by potentiation of tonic inhibition.

AP-like neurosteroids are powerful anticonvulsants [5]. Neurosteroids protect against seizures induced by GABA-A receptor antagonists, including pentylenetetrazol and bicuculline, and are effective against pilocarpine-induced limbic seizures and seizures in kindled animals. Neurosteroids are inactive or only weakly active against seizures elicited by maximal electroshock. In addition, neurosteroids are also highly effective in suppressing seizures due to the withdrawal of GABA-A receptor modulators including neurosteroids and benzodiazepines, as well as other types of agents such as ethanol and cocaine [42,43]. Moreover, neurosteroid exposure leads to cross-tolerance for the anticonvulsant activity of benzodiazepines [44]. In addition to anticonvulsant activity, there is emerging evidence that endogenous neurosteroids play a role in regulating epileptogenesis [27,45,46]. Exogenous treatment with neurosteroids or progesterone has also been reported to delay the occurrence of epileptogenesis. Indeed, progesterone has been shown to retard epileptogenesis in kindling models, even at doses that do not affect seizure expression [27]. Overall, neurosteroids are more robust anticonvulsants than benzodiazepines.

Potential mechanisms of catamenial seizures

Endogenous neurosteroids may play a role in catamenial seizure susceptibility in women with epilepsy. When neurosteroid levels fluctuate, loss of seizure control can occur. Neurosteroids have been implicated in perimenstrual seizure exacerbations in women with a normal menstrual cycle. It is hypothesized that the withdrawal of progesterone-derived neurosteroids leads to enhanced excitability predisposing to seizures [7].

In addition, plasticity in GABA-A receptor subunits could play a role in the enhanced seizure susceptibility in perimenstrual catamenial epilepsy. Animal studies have shown that prolonged exposure to AP followed by withdrawal, such as that which occurs during menstruation, causes a marked increase in expression of the α4 subunit, a key subunit linked to enhanced neuronal excitability, seizure susceptibility, and benzodiazepine resistance [47,48]. Overall, these neuroendocrine changes can result in reduced inhibition resulting in enhanced excitability that, among other effects, predisposes to seizures. In women with epilepsy, finasteride therapy has led to an increase in seizure frequency and severity [49], suggesting that endogenous neurosteroids do modulate seizure susceptibility.

We have developed a rodent model of perimenstrual catamenial epilepsy [50,51]. Withdrawal of neurosteroids led to a decreased seizure threshold and increased seizure activity [50]. In epileptic animals, neurosteroid withdrawal was associated with a marked increase in seizure frequency. The neurosteroid withdrawal model of catamenial epilepsy was used to investigate therapies for perimenstrual catamenial epilepsy [43,44]. A key result is that conventional antiepileptic drugs, including benzodiazepines and valproate, are less potent in protecting against seizures during the period of enhanced seizure susceptibility following neurosteroid withdrawal. This pharmacoresistance appears to mimic the situation in women with catamenial epilepsy where breakthrough seizures occur despite treatment with antiepileptic drugs. In contrast to the results with conventional antiepileptic drugs, neurosteroids including AP were found to have enhanced activity in the catamenial epilepsy model [43]. This suggested a "neurosteroid replacement" approach to treat catamenial seizure exacerbations [52]. A neurosteroid could be administered in a "pulse" prior to menstruation and then withdrawn, or continuously administered throughout the month. The neurosteroid would be administered at low doses to avoid sedative side effects. Such low doses are expected to contribute little anticonvulsant activity during most of the menstrual cycle, but may prevent the occurrence of perimenstrual catamenial seizures.

In addition, the structure of the extrasynaptic GABA-A receptor undergoes drastic alterations due to changing levels of progesterone during the ovarian cycle. Recent studies in animals have demonstrated profound changes in hippocampal GABA-A receptor subunit expression during different phases of the estrous cycle [43,53]. During the late diestrous phase (associated with high progesterone levels), expression of δ-subunit-containing GABA-A receptors was elevated, which was associated with an increase in tonic inhibition and diminished seizure susceptibility in mice. During the phase of estrus (associated with low progesterone levels), tonic inhibition was reduced by 50% with corresponding increases in both seizure susceptibility and anxiety behavior in mice. These cyclic alterations in the δ subunit are also observed following exogenous progesterone treatment in ovariectomized female mice [54]. Unlike the phasic inhibition mediated by γ-subunit-containing GABA-A receptors, the δ-subunit-containing GABA-A receptors are highly sensitive to neurosteroids. Susceptibility to epileptogenesis is lower at diestrous than at estrus. These findings are consistent with the possibility that the abundance of extrasynaptic δ-subunit-containing GABA-A receptors is increased during diestrous, likely due to elevated neurosteroids, and thereby contribute to AP-sensitive GABAergic currents in the hippocampus. It is suggested that deficiencies in regulatory mechanisms controlling normal cycling of δ-subunit-containing GABA-A receptors in the hippocampus could be a potential molecular mechanism for catamenial seizures. Thus, the δ-subunit-containing GABA-A receptor is an important target for developing specific treatments for catamenial epilepsy.

  The overall potential mechanisms of catamenial seizure patterns are summarized in Table 3.2 [7]. Perimenstrual type (C1) occurs in women with ovulatory cycles, possibly due to a sharp decline ("withdrawal") in the serum level of progesterone and consequently of the level of progesterone-derived anticonvulsant neurosteroids in the brain around the perimenstrual period. The ratio of estradiol to neurosteroid is highest during menstruation. Because neurosteroid potentiates GABA-A receptor-mediated inhibition, the rapid loss of neurosteroid-mediated inhibition, such as that which occurs before, during or after the onset of menses, could exacerbate seizures in many women with catamenial epilepsy. Periovulatory type (C2) occurs in women with ovulatory cycles, possibly due to the estradiol surge just before ovulation, and low neurosteroid levels do not offset the estradiol-induced excitation because the rise of anticonvulsant neurosteroid levels would not occur until after ovulation. The relatively low neurosteroid inhibition and marked estradiol excitation could lead to periovulatory seizures. Inadequate luteal type (C3) occurs in women with anovulatory cycles, possibly due to a loss of neurosteroid-mediated inhibition during the luteal phase for a prolonged time and also due to elevated estrogen levels. Progesterone secretion that occurs normally during the luteal phase is markedly decreased during anovulatory cycles, resulting in abnormally low levels of neurosteroid in the brain.

Progesterone therapy for catamenial epilepsy

A small number of hormonal treatment trials have been carried out in women with epilepsy. These trials can be divided into two categories: (i) hormonal suppression and (ii) cyclic progesterone supplementation. Suppression of ovarian hormonal secretion has been accomplished by treatment with intramuscular depomedroxyprogesterone. This strategy is less widely acceptable for reproductive reasons.

Progesterone therapy represents a potential hormonal approach for the treatment of catamenial epilepsy. In clinical studies progesterone has been found to reduce seizures [55,56]. Previous open-label studies suggest that the cyclic administration of adjunctive natural progesterone supplement may lessen seizure frequency by over 50% in the majority of women with catamenially exacerbated intractable seizures [56,57]. Oral synthetic progestins, in contrast, have not shown significant efficacy. In general, progesterone should be administered during the entire second half of the menstrual cycle and tapered gradually, as it is believed that abrupt discontinuation can result in rebound seizure exacerbation.

A NIH-sponsored clinical study to assess progesterone treatment of intractable seizures in women with partial epilepsy was recently completed [58]. This randomized, double-blind, placebo-controlled, phase III, multicenter clinical trial compared the efficacy and safety of adjunctive cyclic natural progesterone therapy with placebo treatment of intractable seizures in 294 subjects randomized 2 : 1 to progesterone or placebo, stratified by catamenial and noncatamenial status. It compared treatments on proportions of ≥50% responders and changes in seizure frequency from three baselines to three treated menstrual cycles. The results indicate that there was no significant difference in proportions of responders between progesterone and placebo in the catamenial and noncatamenial patients. However, a post-hoc analysis found a significantly higher responder rate in women with perimenstrual seizure exacerbation (C1). Reductions in seizure frequency correlated with increasing C1 levels for progesterone but not placebo, progressing from 26 to 71% for progesterone and from 25 to 26% for placebo. These findings suggest that progesterone may provide a clinically important benefit for a subset of women with perimenstrual catamenial epilepsy. The mechanisms underlying the lack of progesterone effect on overall seizure frequency remains unclear. The dramatic response of progesterone, which is a neurosteroid precursor, in women with perimenstrual catamenial epilepsy is attributable to the unique neurosteroid sensitivity of perimenstrual catamenial seizures [7].

Novel treatments for catamenial epilepsy

Although progesterone therapy is beneficial in perimenstrual catamenial epilepsy, it may be associated with hormonal side effects. Neurosteroids that are devoid of hormonal side effects represent a rational treatment strategy for perimenstrual catamenial epilepsy. However, natural neurosteroids such as AP have severe limitations because they have a short half-life, are orally inactive, and may produce hormonal effects due to their metabolism to hormonally active compounds. Synthetic analogs of neurosteroids may overcome these obstacles and side effects associated with natural progesterone therapy. Neurosteroids seem to be the most direct approach to the treatment of catamenial epilepsy, but there are only limited anecdotal data available to support their use [59]. Despite intense research on neurosteroids, there is no neurosteroid-based drug available for patients. Ganaxolone, the synthetic analog of AP, is the only neurosteroid that has been evaluated for the treatment of epilepsy in humans [60,61]. Ganaxolone has similar pharmacological properties to the natural neurosteroids such as AP. It has protective activity in diverse rodent seizure models [42,62]. Ganaxolone has been tested in various clinical trials to assess efficacy in the treatment of epilepsy. A phase IIB clinical trial of ganaxolone showed a significant reduction in seizure frequency. However, there are limited data supporting the efficacy of ganaxolone in the treatment of catamenial epilepsy.

Conclusions

Although ovarian hormones play a central role, the exact cause of catamenial epilepsy is unknown. Experimental studies to this point have indicated a clear role for estrogen, progesterone and endogenous neurosteroids in the pathophysiology of catamenial epilepsy. Although there are several forms of catamenial epilepsy, neurosteroids have been implicated only in the seizure exacerbations that occur around the perimenstrual period. It is hypothesized that the withdrawal of progesterone-derived neurosteroids leads to enhanced neuronal excitability predisposing to seizures. In addition to neurosteroid fluctuations, there is emerging evidence that plasticity in GABA-A receptor subunits could play a role in the enhanced seizure susceptibility in catamenial epilepsy. Animal studies have shown that prolonged exposure to AP followed by withdrawal, such as that which occurs during menstruation, causes a marked increase in expression of the extrasynaptic $\alpha 4$ and δ subunits, which are linked to enhanced neuronal excitability, seizure susceptibility, and benzodiazepine resistance. Overall, these neuroendocrine changes can result in reduced inhibition resulting in enhanced excitability that, among other effects, predisposes to catamenial seizures.

Acknowledgments

The original research described in this chapter was supported in part by NIH grants NS051398, NS052158 and NS071597 (to D.S.R.).

Key summary points

- Neurosteroids are steroids that rapidly alter neuronal excitability through non-genomic mechanisms.

- Neurosteroids rapidly alter neuronal excitability through direct interaction with GABA-A receptors, which are the major receptors for the inhibitory neurotransmitter GABA.

- The GABA-A receptor binding sites for neurosteroids are distinct from the recognition sites for GABA, benzodiazepines, and barbiturates.

- Plasticity in GABA-A receptor subunits, influenced by the cyclic hormonal mileu, could play a role in the occurrence of perimenstrual catamenial epilepsy.

- Prolonged allopregnanolone exposure leads to an increase in the expression of GABA-A receptor extrasynaptic $\alpha 4$ and δ-subunits, which is associated with increased seizure susceptibility and benzodiazepine resistance.

- A leading hypothesis for the mechanism of premenstrual catamenial seizure occurrence in women with epilepsy is the cyclic withdrawal of progesterone-derived neurosteroids leading to enhanced neuronal excitability.

References

1 Baulieu E-E. Steroid hormones in the brain: several mechanisms? In: Fuxe F, Gustafsson JA, Wetterberg L (eds) *Steroid Hormone Regulation of the Brain*. Oxford: Pergamon Press, 1981:3–14.

2 Selye H. Anesthetics of steroid hormones. *Proc Soc Exp Biol Med* 1941;46:116–121.

3 Harrison NL, Simmonds MA. Modulation of the GABA receptor complex by a steroid anaesthetic. *Brain Res* 1984;323:287–292.

4 Majewska MD, Harrison NL, Schwartz RD, Barker JL, Paul SM. Steroid hormone metabolites are barbiturate-like modulators of the GABA receptor. *Science* 1986;232:1004–1007.

5 Reddy DS. Role of anticonvulsant and antiepileptogenic neurosteroids in the pathophysiology and treatment of epilepsy. *Front Endocrinol* 2011;2:38.

6 Reddy DS, Jian K. The testosterone-derived neurosteroid androstanediol is a positive allosteric modulator of $GABA_A$ receptors. *J Pharmacol Exp Ther* 2010;334:1031–1041.

7 Reddy DS. The role of neurosteroids in the pathophysiology and treatment of catamenial epilepsy. *Epilepsy Res* 2009;85:1–30.

8 Herzog AG, Harden CL, Liporace J *et al*. Frequency of catamenial seizure exacerbation in women with localization-related epilepsy. *Ann Neurol* 2004;56:431–434.

9 Bazan AC, Montenegro MA, Cendes F, Min LL, Guerreiro CA. Menstrual cycle worsening of epileptic seizures in women with symptomatic focal epilepsy. *Arg Neuro-Psiquiatria* 2005;63(3B):751–756.

10 Gilad R, Sadeh M, Rapoport A, Dabby R, Lampl Y. Lamotrigine and catamenial epilepsy. *Seizure* 2008;17:531–534.

11 Herzog AG, Klein P, Ransil BJ. Three patterns of catamenial epilepsy. *Epilepsia* 1997;38:1082–1088.

12 Herzog AG, Fowler KM. Sensitivity and specificity of the association between catamenial seizure patterns and ovulation. *Neurology* 2008;70:486–487.

13 Quigg M, Smithson SD, Fowler KM, Sursal T, Herzog AG. NIH Progesterone Trial Study Group: laterality and location influence catamenial seizure expression in women with partial epilepsy. *Neurology* 2009;73:223–227.

14 Bauer J, Burr W, Elger CE. Seizure occurrence during ovulatory and anovulatory cycles in patients with temporal lobe epilepsy: a prospective study. *Eur J Neurol* 1998;5:83–88.

15 Bauer J. Interactions between hormones and epilepsy in female patients. *Epilepsia* 2001;42(Suppl 3):20–22.

16 Pack AM, Reddy DS, Duncan S, Herzog A. Neuroendocrinological aspects of epilepsy: important issues and trends in future research. *Epilepsy Behav* 2011;22:94–102.

17 Velíšková J. Estrogens and epilepsy: why are we so excited? *Neuroscientist* 2007;13: 77–88.

18 Reibel S, André V, Chassagnon S *et al.* Neuroprotective effects of chronic estradiol benzoate treatment on hippocampal cell loss induced by status epilepticus in the female rat. *Neurosci Lett* 2000;281:79–82.

19 Velíšková J, Velisek L, Galanopoulou AS, Sperber EF. Neuroprotective effects of estrogens on hippocampal cells in adult female rats after status epilepticus. *Epilepsia* 2000;41(Suppl 6):S30–S35.

20 Logothetis J, Harner R, Morrel F. The role of estrogens in catamenial exacerbation of epilepsy. *Neurology* 1959;9:352–360.

21 Bäckström T. Epileptic seizures in women related to plasma estrogen and P during the menstrual cycle. *Acta Neurol Scand* 1976;54:321–347.

22 Bonuccelli U, Melis GB, Paoletti AM, Fioretti P, Murri L, Muratorio A. Unbalanced progesterone and estradiol secretion in catamenial epilepsy. *Epilepsy Res* 1989;3:100–106.

23 Jacono JJ, Robinson J. The effects of estrogen, progesterone, and ionized calcium on seizures during the menstrual cycle in epileptic women. *Epilepsia* 1987;28:571–577.

24 Craig CR. Anticonvulsant activity of steroids: separability of anticonvulsant from hormonal effects. *J Pharmacol Exp Ther* 1966;153:337–343.

25 Landgren S, Bäckström T, Kalistratov G. The effect of progesterone on the spontaneous interictal spike evoked by the application of penicillin to the cat's cerebral cortex. *J Neurol Sci* 1978;36:119–133.

26 Reddy DS, Castaneda DC, O'Malley BW, Rogawski MA. Anticonvulsant activity of progesterone and neurosteroids in progesterone receptor knockout mice. *J Pharmacol Exp Ther* 2004;310:230–239.

27 Reddy DS, Gangisetty O, Briyal S. Disease-modifying activity of progesterone in the hippocampus kindling model of epileptogenesis. *Neuropharmacology* 2010;59:573–581.

28 Tuveri A, Paoletti AM, Orrù M *et al.* Reduced serum level of THDOC, an anticonvulsant steroid, in women with perimenstrual catamenial epilepsy. *Epilepsia* 2008;49:1221–1229.

29 El-Khayat HA, Soliman NA, Tomoum HY, Omran MA, El-Wakad AS, Shatla RH. Reproductive hormonal changes and catamenial pattern in adolescent females with epilepsy. *Epilepsia* 2008;49:1619–1626.

30 Agís-Balboa RC, Pinna G, Zhubi A *et al.* Characterization of brain neurons that express enzymes mediating neurosteroid biosynthesis. *Proc Natl Acad Sci USA* 2006;103:14602–14607.

31 Do Rego JL, Seong JY, Burel D *et al.* Neurosteroid biosynthesis: enzymatic pathways and neuroendocrine regulation by neurotransmitters and neuropeptides. *Front Neuroendocrinol* 2009;30:259–301.

32 Rupprecht R, Papadopoulos V, Rammes G *et al.* Translocator protein (18 kDa) (TSPO) as a therapeutic target for neurological and psychiatric disorders. *Nat Rev Drug Discov* 2010;9:971–988.

33 Hosie AD, Wilkins ME, da Silva HMA, Smart TG. Endogenous neurosteroids regulate $GABA_A$ receptors through two discrete transmembrane sites. *Nature* 2006;444: 486–489.

34 Hosie AM, Clarke L, da Silva II, Smart TG. Conserved site for neurosteroid modulation of $GABA_A$ receptors. *Neuropharmacology* 2009;56:149–154.

35 Hosie AM, Wilkins ME, Smart TG. Neurosteroid binding sites on GABA$_A$ receptors. *Pharmacol Ther* 2007;116:7–19.

36 Harrison NL, Majewska MD, Harrington JW, Barker JL. Structure–activity relationships for steroid interactions with the γ-aminobutyric acid$_A$ receptor complex. *J Pharmacol Exp Ther* 1987;241:346–353.

37 Reddy DS, Rogawski MA. Stress-induced deoxycorticosterone-derived neuroactive steroids modulates GABA$_A$ receptor function and seizure susceptibility. *J Neurosci* 2002;42:3795–3805.

38 Chisari M, Eisenman LN, Covey DF, Mennerick S, Zorumski CF. The sticky issue of neurosteroids and GABA$_A$ receptors. *Trends Neurosci* 2010;33:299–306.

39 Chisari M, Eisenman LN, Krishnan K *et al*. The influence of neuroactive steroid lipophilicity on GABA$_A$ receptor modulation: evidence for a low-affinity interaction. *J Neurophysiol* 2009;102:1254–1264.

40 Wohlfarth KM, Bianchi MT, Macdonald RL. Enhanced neurosteroid potentiation of ternary GABA$_A$ receptors containing the δ subunit. *J Neurosci* 2002;22:1541–1549.

41 Belelli D, Casula A, Ling AL, Lambert JJ. The influence of subunit composition on the interaction of neurosteroids with GABA$_A$ receptors. *Neuropharmacology* 2002;43:651–661.

42 Devaud LL, Purdy RH, Finn DA, Morrow AL. Sensitization of γ-aminobutyric acid$_A$ receptors to neuroactive steroids in rats during ethanol withdrawal. *J Pharmacol Exp Ther* 1996;278:510–517.

43 Reddy DS, Rogawski MA. Enhanced anticonvulsant activity of neuroactive steroids in a rat model of catamenial epilepsy. *Epilepsia* 2001;42:303–310.

44 Reddy DS, Rogawski MA. Enhanced anticonvulsant activity of ganaxolone after neurosteroid withdrawal in a rat model of catamenial epilepsy. *J Pharmacol Exp Ther* 2000;294:909–915.

45 Biagini G, Baldelli E, Longo D *et al*. Endogenous neurosteroids modulate epileptogenesis in a model of temporal lobe epilepsy. *Exp Neurol* 2006;201:519–524.

46 Biagini G, Longo D, Baldelli E *et al*. Neurosteroids and epileptogenesis in the pilocarpine model: evidence for a relationship between P450scc induction and length of the latent period. *Epilepsia* 2009;50(Suppl 1):53–58.

47 Smith SS, Shen H, Gong QH, Zhou X. Neurosteroid regulation of GABA-A receptors: focus on the alpha4 and delta subunits. *Pharmacol Ther* 2007;116:58–76.

48 Gangisetty O, Reddy DS. Neurosteroid withdrawal regulates GABA$_A$ receptor α$_4$-subunit expression and seizure susceptibility by activation of progesterone receptor-independent early growth response factor-3 pathway. *Neuroscience* 2010;170:865–880.

49 Herzog AG, Frye CA. Seizure exacerbation associated with inhibition of progesterone metabolism. *Ann Neurol* 2003;53:390–391.

50 Reddy DS, Kim HY, Rogawski MA. Neurosteroid withdrawal model of perimenstrual catamenial epilepsy. *Epilepsia* 2001;42:328–336.

51 Reddy DS, Zeng YC. Effect of neurosteroid withdrawal on spontaneous recurrent seizures in a rat model of catamenial epilepsy. *FASEB J* 2007;21:A1179.

52 Reddy DS, Rogawski MA. Neurosteroid replacement therapy for catamenial epilepsy. *Neurotherapeutics* 2009;6:392–401.

53 Maguire JL, Stell BM, Rafizadeh M, Mody I. Ovarian cycle-linked changes in GABA$_A$ receptors mediating tonic inhibition alter seizure susceptibility and anxiety. *Nat Neurosci* 2005;8:797–804.

54 Maguire J, Mody I. Neurosteroid synthesis-mediated regulation of GABA-A receptors: relevance to the ovarian cycle and stress. *J Neurosci* 2007;27:2155–2162.

55 Bäckström T, Zetterlund B, Blom S, Romano M. Effect of intravenous progesterone infusions on the epileptic discharge frequency in women with partial epilepsy. *Acta Neurol Scand* 1984;69:240–248.

56 Herzog AG. Progesterone therapy in women with epilepsy: a 3-year follow-up. *Neurology* 1999;52:1917–1918.

57 Herzog AG. Progesterone therapy in women with complex partial and secondary generalized seizures. *Neurology* 1995;45:1600–1662.

58 Herzog, AG, Fowler KM, Smithson SD *et al*. Progesterone versus placebo therapy for women with epilepsy: a randomized clinical trial. *Neurology* 2012;78:1959–1966.

59 McAuley JW, Reeves AL, Flyak J, Monaghan EP, Data J. A pilot study of the neurosteroid ganaxolone in catamenial epilepsy: clinical experience in two patients. *Epilepsia* 2001;42(Suppl 7):85 (Abstract 1.267).

60 Reddy DS, Woodward R. Ganaxolone: a prospective overview. *Drugs Future* 2004;29:227–242.

61 Rogawski MA, Nohria V, Tsai J, Shaw K, Farfel G, Pieribone VA. Ganaxolone. In: Bialer M, Johannessen SI, Levy RH, Perucca E, Tomson T, White HS. Progress report on new antiepileptic drugs: a summary of the Tenth Eilat Conference (EILAT X). *Epilepsy Res* 2010;92:89–124.

62 Reddy DS, Rogawski MA. Ganaxolone suppression of behavioral and electrographic seizures in the mouse amygdala kindling model. *Epilepsy Res* 2010;89:254–260.

Conflict of Interest Statement

The author declares that the research was conducted in the absence of any commercial or financial relationships that could be construed as a potential conflict of interest.

CHAPTER 4

Catamenial Epilepsy

Erik Taubøll, Line S. Røste and Sigrid Svalheim

Department of Neurology, Oslo University Hospital – Rikshospitalet, Oslo, Norway

---

Case history: *The patient is 55 years old, with epilepsy since the age of 10. She has one adult son. Her main seizure type is complex partial seizures. Previously seizures were occasionally generalized. Seizure frequency has been relatively stable, with two to six seizures per month. A catamenial pattern was first detected in her late teens. Diaries of seizure frequency from childhood and early teens are not available. Between1989 and 1990, she participated in a study on temporal distribution of seizures and was monitored for 323 days (ref. 1, case 10). Approximately 90% of seizures occurred in the premenstrual and menstrual phases, with a somewhat higher frequency premenstrually (Figure 4.1). This pattern has continued, but become less obvious. She has tried several antiepileptic drugs (AEDs) like carbamazepine, phenytoin, valproate, levetiracetam, lamotrigine, topiramate, and clobazam. None of these have affected seizure frequency significantly, nor altered the cyclic pattern. The rhythmic seizure pattern continued during the first half of her pregnancy. For catamenial epilepsy, she has tried acetazolamide 1000mg/day, starting 7 days before menstruation until the third day of the cycle. This had some effect, but did not result in seizure freedom and caused side effects. Cyclic dosing of clobazam had no obvious effect, but as her menstrual cycles were irregular, intermittent treatment was difficult. Medroxyprogesterone acetate (MPA) was tried over a year at a dose that stopped menstrual bleeding. This resulted in the seizures occurring more randomly, which the patient disliked. Seizure frequency has declined since menopause (3 years ago), but continue to occur.*

Introduction to the field

In both men and women with epilepsy, most seizures do not occur randomly [1]. The most frequently encountered pattern is seizure clustering [1,2]. Studies on seizure patterns may elucidate possible underlying mechanisms for seizure precipitation, such as an association to the menstrual cycle. Knowledge on the nonrandom distribution of seizures is also important when evaluating the effect of treatment regimens.

Epilepsy in Women, First Edition. Edited by Cynthia L. Harden, Sanjeev V. Thomas and Torbjörn Tomson.

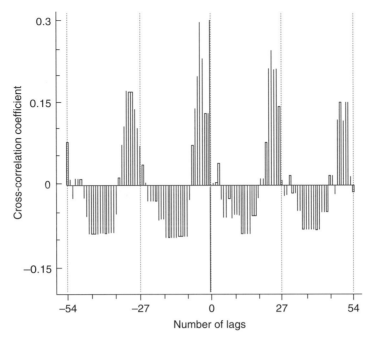

Figure 4.1 Cross-correlogram between the menstrual cycle and seizure occurrence in our patient. Note the local positive peaks occurring about every 4 weeks, indicating a high incidence of co-occurrence of seizures and menstruation. (Published with permission from Taubøll E, Lundervold A, Gjerstad L. Temporal distribution of seizures in epilepsy. *Epilepsy Research* 1991;8:153–155.)

The idea that epileptic seizures in women may be related to their menstrual cycles is at least as old as Hippocrates, who said "cessation of the menstrual flux is the cause of seizures" [3]. A more thorough analysis of the problem came with Gowers' study from 1885 [4]. Among 82 women with epilepsy, a relationship between menstruation and seizure occurrence was observed in 46, with increased seizure frequency mainly observed during the premenstrual and menstrual periods. This was subsequently confirmed in several other studies. In one of the most extensively documented series [5], 50 institutionalized women with generalized tonic–clonic seizures were studied; seizure exacerbation in relation to menstruation was demonstrated in 72%. However, other studies have not confirmed these findings. Binnie *et al.* [6] did not detect a relationship between menstruation and seizure frequency in 14 patients with partial epilepsy. Similarly, a statistical analysis of seizure occurrence in 15 female patients did not demonstrate that seizure cycle was associated with menses [7]. Further, in a study of over 300 patients, the mere existence of catamenial epilepsy was denoted a myth as late as 1989 [8]. These inconsistencies can be explained by several factors, including patient aspects (e.g., reliability of patients and their seizure diaries), large individual variations, differences in phase preferences, and changes in medication. Different definitions of catamenial epilepsy also add to the varied results.

Background and important details

The term "catamenial epilepsy" describes seizure clustering in alignment with the menstrual cycle. Catamenial epilepsy has been reported to occur in as few as 10% of patients [9] to over 70% [1,5]. This wide range mainly reflects the use of very different definitions of catamenial epilepsy, from the requirement that more than 75% of all seizures occur during the 10-day period around menstruation, to the observance of a significant increase in seizure frequency in relation to menstruation without specification of magnitude of change. Thus, there is a clear need for a unifying definition. Before the prevalence of catamenial epilepsy can be determined, the different patterns of seizure exacerbation must first be defined. Secondly, the degree of increase in seizure frequency that is clinically relevant during the selected cycle phase must be agreed.

Herzog and colleagues [10,11] have presented evidence for at least three distinct patterns of catamenial epilepsy (Figure 4.2). The first two patterns account for ovulatory cycles, called perimenstrual (C1) and periovulatory (C2), and the third for anovulatory cycles, called luteal (C3) (Figure 4.2). The patterns of catamenial epilepsy in the individual patient can be determined using a detailed diary of seizures and menses, and with a mid-luteal phase serum progesterone measurement used to distinguish between normal and inadequate luteal phase.

The degree of seizure exacerbation that should be considered sufficient for a diagnosis of catamenial epilepsy, along with clinical relevance, has been controversial. Again individual factors, seizure type, overall seizure frequency, etc., are all of importance. Herzog *et al.* [10,12] proposed a doubling in daily seizure frequency during the phases of exacerbation, relative to baseline phases. Using this criterion, approximately one-third of women with intractable partial epilepsy can be diagnosed as having catamenial epilepsy. We suggest that all studies should use this definition in order to facilitate comparison of results. By far the most common pattern of catamenial epilepsy is the premenstrual type. Catamenial epilepsy occurs with all seizure types and epilepsy syndromes, including idiopathic, cryptogenic, or symptomatic epilepsy [13–16].

All types of AEDs have been used for treatment of catamenial epilepsy. Some AEDs are enzyme inducers, sharing some metabolic pathways with steroid hormones. However, specific patterns between individual drugs and treatment responses have not been unequivocally demonstrated. Since many patients, as in our case, continue to suffer seizures despite many years of different AED treatments, catamenial epilepsy can be considered a form of pharmacoresistant epilepsy. In some patients, seizures only remain in certain phases of the cycle and could thus be designated state-dependent pharmacoresistant epilepsy.

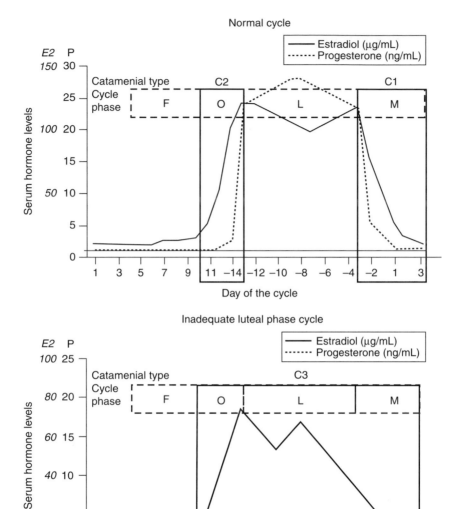

Figure 4.2 Three patterns of catamenial epilepsy: perimenstrual (C1) and periovulatory (C2) exacerbations during normal ovulatory cycles, and entire second half of the cycle (C3) exacerbation during inadequate luteal phase cycles, where day 1 is the first day of menstrual flow and day 14 is the day of ovulation. (Published with permission from Herzog AG. Catamenial epilepsy: definition, prevalence, pathophysiology and treatment. *Seizure* 2008;17:151–159.)

Pathophysiology

The exact causes of catamenial epilepsy are still unclear. To date, there is no evidence that a genetic component is responsible for some women developing catamenial epilepsy. Mechanisms that are potentially involved include fluctuations in AED concentrations and cyclic alterations in reproductive steroid hormones.

Fluctuations in AED concentrations

An association between menstruation and seizures was first described by Hippocrates, and the first systematic reports on catamenial epilepsy were published in the late eighteenth century [4], both well before the era of AEDs. Thus, fluctuations in AED concentrations can, at most, be a contributing factor. There is currently no evidence supporting the hypothesis that cyclic changes in concentrations of regularly used AEDs play any role in catamenial seizure exacerbation. However, it is nevertheless clear that there is an interaction between several AEDs and reproductive steroid hormones. Some enzyme-inducing AEDs can enhance the metabolism of steroid hormones. They also increase sex hormone-binding globulin, thereby further reducing bioactive steroid concentrations. These factors could, theoretically, reduce the effect of cyclic hormonal changes, but this has not been shown to be important for catamenial epilepsy in clinical studies. High concentrations of steroid hormones, especially estrogen, decrease lamotrigine concentrations by 31% in the luteal phase of the menstrual cycle [17], which should, theoretically, worsen catamenial epilepsy. Again, such an association has not been demonstrated. On the contrary, a positive effect of lamotrigine in catamenial epilepsy has been reported in a few cases [18]. Valproate concentrations do not seem to vary during the menstrual cycle [17].

Role of reproductive steroid hormones

There is compelling evidence that reproductive steroids play an important role in the pathophysiology of catamenial epilepsy. Steroids act in the brain by direct and immediate membrane-mediated effects, but also through genomically mediated effects developing over time.

There are three biologically active forms of estrogens: estradiol, estrone, and estriol. For catamenial epilepsy, estradiol is the important. Estradiol exists as two isomers, 17α-estradiol and 17β-estradiol, with the latter the major bioactive form in menstruating women. Estrone is the major form in postmenopausal women, while estriol dominates in pregnancy; both are of minor, if any, importance for catamenial epilepsy. The excitatory effect of estrogens was convincingly demonstrated in 1959 by Logothetis *et al.* [19] who intravenously infused estrogen into women with epilepsy, leading to seizures and even status epilepticus. The excitatory effects of estrogens are related to a direct membrane effect, augmenting *N*-methyl-D-aspartate (NMDA)-mediated glutamate receptor activity, but also to genomically related mechanisms affecting neuronal plasticity. Estrogens increase the density of spines and excitatory NMDA receptor-containing synapses on the apical hippocampal dendrites in CA1 [20], and reduce γ-aminobutyric acid (GABA) synthesis by decreasing glutamic acid decarboxylase activity (see refs 11 and 13 for extensive reviews).

Progesterone and its 3α-hydroxylated metabolites, particularly allopregnanolone (3α-hydroxy-5α-pregnan-20-one), exert strong inhibitory effects on neuronal excitability, through direct membrane effects but also via genomic effects. The antiseizure effect of progesterone was clinically demonstrated by Bäckström *et al.* [21], who showed a reduction in spike frequency when women with epilepsy were infused with progesterone. The inhibitory effect of progesterone and its metabolites have been confirmed in several *in vitro* and *in vivo* studies [22,23]. These acute effects are primarily due to potentiation of a GABA-A-mediated chloride influx. In addition, other long-term genomic effects develop, such as fewer estrogen receptors and less dendritic spines and excitatory synapses, faster than with simple withdrawal of estrogen, counteracting the stimulatory effects of estradiol [20]. Progesterone may also regulate subtype composition of GABA-A receptors, thereby modulating their sensitivity to GABA and other pharmacological agents [24].

In patients with catamenial epilepsy, seizure frequency appears to be related to the estrogen to progesterone (E/P) ratio. This was shown by Bäckström [15], who found a positive correlation between secondary generalized seizures and the mean E/P ratio in ovulatory cycles, and also a negative correlation with plasma progesterone levels. It was recently found that in anovulatory cycles secondary generalized seizures, rather than complex or simple partial seizures, were higher than in ovulatory cycles, and that this could be related to a proportional increase in E/P ratio [16]. In patients with catamenial epilepsy, estradiol concentrations are similar to those in control subjects during the cycle [13,25]. However, progesterone levels seem lower, at least in the mid-luteal phase. Consequently, the E/P ratio is reduced. Reduced E/P ratio occurs perimenstrually in patients with perimenstrual catamenial epilepsy. These results illustrate that an increased E/P ratio is essential for developing a catamenial seizure pattern. In addition to the ratio itself, it has been proposed that premenstrual seizure exacerbation is also related to the rate of decline of progesterone, inducing a sort of withdrawal syndrome (see ref. 14 for review).

Treatment

There is no established treatment for catamenial epilepsy. Treatment strategies can be hormonal or nonhormonal. Hormonal treatment appears to be effective in some patients.

Hormonal treatment
Cyclic progesterone treatment

Treatment with progestogens can be either cyclic or chronic. Cyclic treatment has been given with natural progesterone, while synthetic progestins like MPA have been used for chronic treatment (for reviews, see refs 11, 25 and 26).

The first study of cyclic progesterone therapy included eight women with complex partial seizures and anovulatory cycles [27]. Progesterone was administered as vaginal suppositories during the premenstrual phase or entire second half of the cycle, in doses of 100–200 mg three times per day (t.i.d.). Average monthly seizure frequency declined by 68% during the 3-month study period, and six of eight patients improved [27]. Positive effects from intermittent treatment with natural progesterone in the last half of the cycle have since been shown, with a gradual reduction over 3–4 days to avoid withdrawal effects and seizures. Progesterone was administered as lozenges in doses of 100–200 mg t.i.d., with individual adjustment according to progesterone serum concentrations, which were maintained at between 20 and 40 ng/mL [28]. In several patients, treatment remained effective after 3 years [29]. Recently, the first preliminary data from a large National Institutes of Health (NIH)-sponsored phase III study on progesterone treatment in catamenial epilepsy were presented [30]. This randomized, double-blinded, placebo-controlled, multicenter clinical trial compared short-term (3 month) efficacy and safety of cyclic natural progesterone therapy for treating intractable seizures in women with focal onset epilepsy. In this study, 294 subjects were included, randomized 2 : 1 to progesterone or placebo treatment, and stratified by catamenial and noncatamenial status. Progesterone was administered at doses of 200 mg t.i.d. from days 14 to 25, then tapered off with 100 mg t.i.d. on days 26 and 27, and 50 mg t.i.d. on day 28. In patients with catamenial epilepsy, a significant effect of progesterone treatment was only observed in women with the perimenstrual (C1) pattern, and only in those with an approximately threefold increase in perimenstrual seizure frequency. No effect was found in patients with other catamenial seizure patterns.

It seems that progesterone treatment during the whole second half of the cycle is more effective than only during the premenstrual phase, which has also been tried. Whether the positive effect is due to progesterone itself, to its metabolites, or both is currently unresolved. However, addition to progesterone therapy of a 5α-reductase inhibitor like finasteride that blocks transition from progesterone to allopregnanolone results in a marked increase in seizure frequency [31]. This indicates that at least some of the antiseizure effect of progesterone is mediated through its metabolites. The role of progesterone on intracellular receptors has not been elucidated, but is probably of minor importance for treatment of catamenial epilepsy.

Chronic treatment with synthetic progesterone

Chronic treatment has also been tried with the synthetic progestin MPA [32,33], which reduced seizure frequency by 39%. However, no systematic studies have been conducted since these two first early reports. It is reported that for MPA to be effective against seizures, the doses must be high enough to induce amenorrhea.

GnRH analogs and the estrogen inhibitor clomiphene

Endocrine treatment may also involve gonadotropin-releasing hormone (GnRH) analogs and estrogen receptor antagonists. Both are currently highly experimental treatments. GnRH is secreted in a pulsatile fashion and leads to the cyclic release of follicle-stimulating hormone and luteinizing hormone, important for ovulation and a regular menstrual cycle. Using a GnRH inhibitor, the pulsatile pattern is abolished, cyclicity ceases, and a menopause-like state ensues. A few small, open studies using GnRH analogs like goserelin [34] and triptorelin [35] have reported positive results, but these must be replicated in larger studies. The antiestrogen clomiphene (INN clomifene) achieved promising results in one small study [36], but again follow-up studies are lacking.

Ganaxolone

Ganaxolone, a synthetic analog of the endogenous neurosteroid allopregnanolone, is an interesting new AED that induces positive allosteric modulation of GABA-A receptors [14,37]. It has been investigated in several clinical studies and seems to be safe and broad spectrum [27]. In preclinical studies, using a pseudopregnancy model of catamenial epilepsy, it was found that ganaxolone's anticonvulsant potency was actually enhanced in the period following neurosteroid withdrawal, perhaps due to a relative increase in the expression of the neurosteroid-sensitive δ-subunit-containing perisynaptic/extrasynaptic GABA-A receptors [25]. The cyclic changes in GABA receptor subunit composition during the menstrual cycle, with ganaxolone being more effective during periods of seizure exacerbation, may indicate that ganaxalone is especially relevant for treating patients with catamenial epilepsy. Larger clinical studies should explore this further.

Side effects of hormonal treatment

All hormonal treatment has the possibility of inducing side effects, including sedation, depression, breast tenderness, weight gain, and vaginal bleeding. In addition, progesterone can sporadically cause diarrhea, dry mouth, edema, headache, irritability, muscular pain, nausea, cramping, acne, hirsutism, and decreased libido. Serious, but rare, side effects are urticaria, anaphylaxis, stroke, retinal thrombosis, hyperlipidemia, and pulmonary embolism. As for all other pharmacological treatments, side effects must always be balanced against beneficial effects.

Nonhormonal treatment

Nonhormonal treatment of catamenial epilepsy has been generally unsuccessful. Such treatment has addressed either (i) acetazolamide, water and electrolyte balance or (ii) intermittent AED treatment.

Azetazolamide has long been used for treating catamenial epilepsy. It is a potent inhibitor of carbonic anhydrase, and its effect in epilepsy is probably related to production of metabolic acidosis. Although used with some success, tolerance develops after prolonged use. Intermittent treatment with acetazolamide around menstruation has been effective in individual cases, with no tolerance observed, but controlled studies have not been conducted.

Other intermittent drug treatment has also been tried. In one study involving 13 women, clobazam (20–30 mg/day) was administered for 10 days around menstruation [38] and found to be effective in nine of them, although only temporarily for four. Tolerance was not observed, even over 1 year. However, the patients selected for this study had responded favorably to the drug in an earlier short-term, placebo-controlled, cross-over study. The potential of intermittent clobazam treatment has not been studied further.

Intermittent changes in dose of current medication have not been investigated thoroughly. Although large individual variations occur, many patients tolerate a dose alteration of 20–30%, depending on the drug. Thus, for individual patients on different drugs like carbamazepine, valproate and lamotrigine, we have increased dosage intermittently by approximately 30% for a 10-day period around menstruation. Individual cases have been positive, but there has been no systematic documentation of results. Increasing current drug dosages rather than adding a new drug intermittently should be investigated in controlled studies.

A few reports suggest that lamotrigine could be a treatment alternative for patients with catamenial epilepsy [18]. Theoretically, this sounds improbable as the high E/P ratio would normally reduce lamotrigine concentration.

Review of the case: Our case represents both typical and atypical aspects of catamenial epilepsy. Most typical is the seizure type (partial seizures with secondary generalizations) and the premenstrual pattern. Generalizations were too few for statistical evaluation of the difference between secondary generalized and complex partial seizures, with regard to cyclicity. However, all types of seizures can show a catamenial pattern.

Her premenstrual seizure pattern is that which occurs most frequently in catamenial epilepsy, i.e., pattern C1 according to Herzog [11]. Our patient's catamenial seizures were difficult to treat and considered pharmacoresistant. The many different failed treatment strategies also illustrate one problem for these patients, and this is associated with the intermittent treatment approach advocated by several specialists. In our experience, this can be problematic as patients with epilepsy often have irregular menses. Thus intermittent treatment is difficult per se and may result in confusion and disappointment for the patient. Thus, a treatment strategy involving a drug that can also be used regularly would be preferable.

Another aspect of this case, and others in our clinic, is the lack of effect of MPA. Using doses leading to amenorrhea, the results have been disappointing. As early studies were promising, it is surprising that the efficacy of MPA treatment has not been studied further. The tendency of a continuing nonrandom seizure pattern, even in pregnancy, is noteworthy. This challenges the hypothesis that catamenial epilepsy is solely related to hormonal changes. Seizures may vary according to other factors than the menstrual cycle.

Our patient is now menopausal, but still suffers from seizures. There is still some seizure clustering, although not related to menstruation. The role of menopause itself on changes in both seizure pattern and seizure frequency has not been studied in detail and should be addressed in further studies.

Our case illustrates the importance of catamenial epilepsy for life and well-being, as a pharmacoresistant type of epilepsy. Several aspects of catamenial epilepsy are still poorly understood, with regard to both pathophysiology and effective treatment. Further investigations, including randomized studies on different treatment strategies, should be encouraged. Some studies are already in progress, particularly regarding treatment with progesterone, and the results are eagerly awaited.

Key summary points

- Catamenial epilepsy denotes an association between menstrual cycle and seizure frequency.
- The different prevalences reported for catamenial epilepsy are partly due to the many definitions used.
- Catamenial epilepsy should be defined as a doubling in average daily seizure frequency during the phase of exacerbation, relative to baseline phases [10–12].
- With this definition, approximately one-third of women with intractable partial epilepsy would be diagnosed with catamenial epilepsy.
- Catamenial epilepsy occurs with every seizure type and epilepsy syndrome.
- There are three main seizure patterns in catamenial epilepsy: in those with ovulatory cycles, perimenstrual (most common) and periovulatory patterns; in those with inadequate luteal phase, the luteal pattern.

- The exact cause or causes of catamenial epilepsy remain unclear. To date, there is no evidence that a genetic component is responsible for some women developing catamenial epilepsy.

- Potential mechanisms that have been discussed include (i) fluctuations in AED concentrations; (ii) changes in water and electrolyte balance; and (iii) cyclic alterations in reproductive steroid hormones.

- There is compelling evidence that reproductive steroids play an important role in the pathophysiology of catamenial epilepsy; in particular there is an association between seizure frequency and estrogen/progesterone ratio. Brain excitability is elevated by estrogen and depressed by progesterone and its metabolites.

- There is no established treatment for catamenial epilepsy. Treatment strategies are either hormonal or nonhormonal.

- Hormonal treatment, especially cyclic progesterone treatment, has proven effective in some patients. The new AED ganaxolone may provide an alternative treatment option.

- Nonpharmacologic treatment has not been studied in randomized trials, but treatment strategies like acetazolamide, and intermittent AED treatment, particularly with clobazam, has been advocated. Results have not been convincing.

References

1 Taubøll E, Lundervold A, Gjerstad L. Temporal distribution of seizures in epilepsy. *Epilepsy Res* 1991;8:153–165.
2 Almqvist R. The rhythm of epileptic attacks and its relationship to the menstrual cycle. *Acta Psychiatr Neurol Scand Suppl* 1955;105:1–116.
3 Temkin O. *The Falling Sickness*. Baltimore: The Johns Hopkins Press, 1945.
4 Gowers WR. *Epilepsy and Other Chronic Convulsive Diseases. Their Causes, Symptoms, and Treatment*. New York: William Wood, 1885.
5 Laidlaw J. *Catamenial epilepsy*. Lancet 1956;271:1235–1237.
6 Binnie CD, Aarts JHP, Houtkooper MA *et al*. Temporal characteristics of seizures and epileptiform discharges. *Electroencephalogr Clin Neurophysiol* 1984;58:498–505.
7 Milton JG, Gotman J, Remillard GM, Andermann F. Timing of seizure recurrence in adult epileptic patients: a statistical analysis. *Epilepsia* 1987;28:471–478.
8 Newmark ME. Catamenial epilepsy: a neurological myth persisting for more than 100 years. *Epilepsia* 1989;30:704.
9 Duncan S, Read CL, Brodie MJ. How common is catamenial epilepsy? *Epilepsia* 1993;34:827–831.
10 Herzog AG, Klein P, Ransil BJ. Three patterns of catamenial epilepsy. *Epilepsia* 1997;28:1082–1088.
11 Herzog AG. Catamenial epilepsy: definition, prevalence, pathophysiology and treatment. *Seizure* 2008;17:151–159.
12 Herzog AG, Harden CL, Liporace J *et al*. Frequency of catamenial seizure exacerbation in women with localization-related epilepsy. *Ann Neurol* 2004;56:431–434.
13 El-Khayat HA, Soliman NA, Tomoum HY, Omran MA, El-Wakad AS, Shatla RH. Reproductive hormonal changes and catamenial pattern in adolescent females with epilepsy. *Epilepsia* 2008;49:1619–1626.
14 Reddy DS. The role of neurosteroids in the pathophysiology and treatment of catamenial epilepsy. *Epilepsy Res* 2009;85:1–30.

15 Bäckström T. Epileptic seizures in women related to plasma estrogen and progesterone during the menstrual cycle. *Acta Neurol Scand* 1976;54:321–347.

16 Herzog AG, Fowler KM, Sperling MR *et al.* Variation of seizure frequency with ovulatory status of menstrual cycles. *Epilepsia* 2011;52:1843–1848.

17 Herzog AG, Blum AS, Farina EL *et al.* Valproate and lamotrigine level variation with menstrual cycle phase and oral contraceptive use. *Neurology* 2009;72:911–914.

18 Gilad R, Sadeh M, Rapoport A, Dabby R, Lampl Y. Lamotrigine and catamenial epilepsy. *Seizure* 2008;17:531–534.

19 Logothetis J, Harner, Morrell F, Torres F. The role of estrogens in catamenial exacerbation of epilepsy. Neurology 1959;9:352–360.

20 Woolley CS, McEwen BS. Estradiol regulates hippocampal dendritic spine density via an N-methyl-D-aspartate receptor-dependent mechanism. *J Neurosci* 1994;14:7680–7687.

21 Bäckström T, Zetterlund B, Blom S, Romano M. Effects of intravenous progesterone infusions on the epileptic discharge frequency in women with partial epilepsy. *Acta Neurol Scand* 1984;69:240–248.

22 Majewska MD, Harrison NL, Schwartz RD, Barker JL, Paul SM. Steroid hormone metabolites are barbiturate-like modulators of the GABA receptor. *Science* 1986;232:1004–1007.

23 Taubøll E, Lindström S. The effect of progesterone and its metabolite 5α-pregnan-3α-ol-20-one on focal epileptic seizures in the cat's visual cortex *in vivo. Epilepsy Res* 1993;14:17–30.

24 Maguire JL, Stell BM, Rafizadeh M, Mody I. Ovarian cycle-linked changes in GABA(A) receptors mediating tonic inhibition alter seizure susceptibility and anxiety. *Nat Neurosci* 2005;8:797–804.

25 Reddy DS, Rogawski MA. Neurosteroid replacement therapy for catamenial epilepsy. *Neurotherapeutics* 2009;6:392–401.

26 Stevens SJ, Harden CL. Hormonal therapy for epilepsy. *Curr Neurol Neurosci Rep* 2011;11:435–442.

27 Herzog AG. Intermittent progesterone therapy and frequency of complex partial seizures in women with menstrual disorders. *Neurology* 1986;36:1607–1610.

28 Herzog AG. Progesterone therapy in complex partial and secondary generalized seizures. *Neurology* 1995;45:1660–1662.

29 Herzog AG. Progesterone therapy in women with epilepsy: a 3-year follow-up. *Neurology* 1999;52:1917–1918.

30 Herzog AG, Fowler KM, Smithson SD *et al.* Progesterone vs placebo therapy for women with epilepsy: a randomized clinical trial. *Neurology* 2012;78:1959–1966.

31 Herzog AG, Frye CA. Seizure exacerbation associated with inhibition of progesterone metabolism. *Ann Neurol* 2003;53:390–391.

32 Zimmerman AW, Holder DT, Reiter EO, Dekaban AS. Medroxyprogesterone acetate in the treatment of seizures associated with menstruation. *J Pediatr* 1973;83:959–963.

33 Mattson RH, Cramer JA, Caldwell BV, Siconolfi BC. Treatment of seizures with medroxyprogesterone acetate: preliminary report. *Neurology* 1984;34:1255–1258.

34 Haider Y, Barnett DB. Catamenial epilepsy and goserelin. *Lancet* 1991;338:1530.

35 Bauer J, Wildt L, Flügel D, Stefan H. The effect of a synthetic GnRH analogue on catamenial epilepsy: a study in ten patients. *J Neurol* 1992;239:284–286.

36 Herzog AG. Clomiphene therapy in epileptic women with menstrual disorders. *Neurology* 1988;38:432–434.

37 Reddy DS, Woodward R. Ganaxolone: a prospective overview. *Drugs Future* 2004;29:227–242.

38 Feely M, Gibson J. Intermittent clobazam for catamenial epilepsy: tolerance avoided. *J Neurol Neurosurg Psychiatry* 1984;47:1279–1282.

CHAPTER 5

Impact of Epilepsy and AEDs on Reproductive Health

Gerhard Luef

Head of the Epilepsy Study Group, Medical University Innsbruck, Innsbruck, Austria

---

Case history: *A 32-year-old woman with a history of three tonic–clonic seizures that occurred between the ages of 19 and 20 years was referred to the epilepsy outpatient clinic of the Department of Neurology. She had no history of febrile seizures, the scalp EEG showed occasional left temporal slowing, and magnetic resonance imaging (MRI) was normal. Because she was overweight when she was younger, she was started on topiramate 100 mg/day and became free of tonic–clonic seizures. When she planned pregnancy at the age of 29, she asked her gynecologist about the safety of the drug during pregnancy. She also reported abnormal variation in cycle intervals and particularly painful menstrual cycles, with heavy bleeding. When she did not become pregnant within 2 years and the gynecologist diagnosed anovulatory cycles, a possible influence of topiramate on the menstrual cycle was considered.*

The patient reported that she lost weight while taking topiramate, that the drug was well tolerated and that she had had no tonic–clonic seizures for more than 10 years. However, on detailed questioning, she also reported recurrent strange feelings that she had noticed intermittently for more than 15 years. She thought that these sensations occurred usually a few days before or during the first days of her period. She did report it because she thought it was a kind of panic reaction. During admission to the epilepsy monitoring unit for further evaluation of these spells, these strange feelings were found to be simple and complex partial seizures which occurred without reducing the dosage of topiramate. A medication change was undertaken to improve seizure control; topiramate was changed to levetiracetam and the auras and complex partial seizures disappeared and menstrual disorders and ovulation improved.

Background and important details

Epilepsy, antiepileptic drugs (AEDs), and the reproductive system have complex interactions. One of the most dire reproductive problems, reduced fertility, has been reported more frequently in both men and women with epilepsy than in the general population [1,2]. Reproductive endocrine

---

Epilepsy in Women, First Edition. Edited by Cynthia L. Harden, Sanjeev V. Thomas and Torbjörn Tomson.

disorders are more common among patients with epilepsy than among the population in general. These disorders have been attributed both to epilepsy itself and to AEDs. Epidemiologic studies have found that women and men with epilepsy are less likely to have children, a finding that may encompass infertility but likely contributing causes include factors such as avoidance of pregnancy due to epilepsy [1,3,4]. However, women with epilepsy face different issues than do men with epilepsy [5]. Women with epilepsy are at increased risk for reproductive disorders. Reproductive dysfunction is often associated with, and are the consequence of, reproductive endocrine disorders. In women it generally manifests as menstrual disorder, hirsutism, and infertility [6–8], which are also features of polycystic ovary syndrome.

Initially, reproductive endocrine disorders were suggested to be associated with epilepsy itself rather than with the medication. However, in the late 1970s and 1980s serum levels of sex hormone-binding globulin were reported to be elevated in women taking enzyme-inducing drugs for epilepsy. Importantly, Margraf and Dreifuss [9] were the first to report amenorrhea following initiation of therapy with valproate, indicating a drug-induced effect.

There is a mounting literature (experimental and clinical) that has focused on possible pathways underlying the interplay between hormones, epilepsy and AEDs [10]. Nevertheless, extrapolation of animal or experimental data to humans is precarious. In humans the interaction between medication, dosage, seizure control, type of seizure, and patient compliance is complicated. Furthermore, different types of epilepsy (with different ages of onset) require different treatment regimens that influence sex steroid hormones, lipid metabolism, the neuro-cardio-endocrine axis, bone metabolism, and thyroid hormones in a specific manner [11]. It is often difficult to determine whether these abnormalities are due to epilepsy-related hypothalamic–pituitary axis dysfunction or to side effects of the AEDs used. For example, a direct influence of epilepsy on the reproductive endocrine system is reflected by acute changes in prolactin and gonadotropin levels following generalized and partial seizures, suggesting a possible relationship between temporo-limbic epileptiform discharges and particular reproductive endocrine disorders [8,12,13]. There are also important clinical findings which indicate that reproductive endocrine function differs between women with epilepsy and healthy controls and that the laterality and focality of epilepsy may be important determinants of reproductive endocrine function [14]. Unilateral temporo-limbic discharges are associated with laterally differing, consistent, predictable, stochastic directional changes in hormonal secretion at all levels of the reproductive neuroendocrine axis, i.e., hypothalamus, pituitary, and ovary [14]. Postictal hormonal changes are not relevant after a single seizure; however, endocrine dysfunction can follow serial uncontrolled seizures, even unrecognized simple partial seizures [13].

Menstrual disorders

Menstrual disorders can be categorized as amenorrhea (no menses for 6 months), oligomenorrhea (cycle interval >32 days), polymenorrhea (cycle interval <26 days), abnormal variation in cycle interval (>4 days), and menometrorrhagia (heavy menses and bleeding between menses) [15]. Cycle intervals of 26–32 days, rather than the currently popular broader range of 21–35 days, should be considered normal in women with epilepsy because ovulatory rates drop substantially and statistically signi-ficantly (i.e., from >75% to <50%) outside the 26–32 day range [16]. The occurrence of ovulation in this population is an important marker of reproductive health, with the additional consideration that anovulatory cycles are associated with greater seizure frequency [17].

Menstrual disorders are currently estimated to occur in one-third of women with epilepsy compared with 12–14% of women in the general population [15]. More than one-third of cycles in women with localization-related epilepsy are anovulatory, as compared with 8–10% in controls [15–19]. Hypothalamic amenorrhea [i.e., amenorrhea associated with low gonadotropin and estrogen levels and diminished luteinizing hormone (LH) response to gonadotropin-releasing hormone (GnRH) challenge], functional hyperprolactinemia (elevated prolactin levels without identifiable pituitary lesion), and premature menopause (cessation of ovarian function featuring amenorrhea and elevated gonadotropin levels) have been found to be over-represented in women with epilepsy [1,7,14,16,20]. In an investigation of 50 consecutive women with clinical and electroencephalographic features of temporal lobe epilepsy, 28 (56%) had amenorrhea, oligomenorrhea, or abnormally long or short menstrual cycle intervals [7]. Of the 28 women with epilepsy and menstrual disorders, 19 (68%, 38% overall) had readily identifiable reproductive endocrine disorders. The data showed no significant relationship overall between the occurrence of menstrual disorders and the use of AEDs (53% among users vs. 60% among nonusers) and raised the possibility that epilepsy itself may be a factor [7].

As described by Herzog *et al.* [8] in 1986, oligomenorrhea is seen in 20–50% of women with temporal lobe epilepsy receiving AEDs. There is still conflicting evidence as to whether anovulatory cycles are more common with localization-related epilepsy or primary generalized epilepsy [18,21]. Women with idiopathic epilepsy are only 37% as likely as unaffected female siblings to become pregnant. This finding is not attributable to marital rate or to seizure type, age at onset, or family history of epilepsy [22]. In comparison with the general female population, fertility is reduced to 69–85% of the expected number of offspring among married women with epilepsy, primarily temporal lobe epilepsy [1,4].

Polycystic ovary syndrome

The most common reproductive endocrine disorder in women with epilepsy as well as women in the general population is polycystic ovary syndrome (PCOS) [7,16]. PCOS occurs in 10–20% of women with epilepsy compared with 5–6% of women in the general population [1,14,23,24]. This increased rate of occurrence may be of considerable medical significance because PCOS is associated with a higher prevalence of migraine, emotional disorders, diabetes, cardiovascular disease, and female cancers in the general population [24]. PCOS represents the failure of the ovarian follicle to complete normal maturation during the menstrual cycle or a series of cycles, a failure that is perhaps related to the presence of inadequate levels of pituitary follicle-stimulating hormone (FSH), while levels of LH are normal or elevated. These conditions can produce two results. There is failure of ovulation and the partially developed follicle is retained in the ovary in the form of a tiny cyst [14,24]. This partially developed follicle is secretory but deficient in aromatase, the enzyme that converts testosterone to estrogen, and therefore has testosterone as its principal secretory product [16]. Testosterone may increase the positive feedback of estrogen on pituitary LH secretion [25], resulting in increased ovarian steroid secretion which, under these circumstances, may be predominantly testosterone and can result in hyperandrogenism. The testosterone is aromatized in peripheral adipose tissue, generally producing high-normal levels of estrogens that are a major source of the estrogen feedback on the pituitary. The persistent occurrence of such cycles results in hyperandrogenic chronic anovulation, which is currently the simplest and perhaps the most utilitarian definition of PCOS [16,24].

Effect of epilepsy on hypothalamo-pituitary axis

The brain controls reproductive function primarily through hypothalamic regulation of pituitary secretion [26]. Regions of the hypothalamus that are involved in the regulation, production, and secretion of GnRH receive extensive direct connections from the cerebral hemispheres, especially from temporo-limbic structures that are commonly involved in epilepsy, and most notably from the amygdala. Significant relationships have been uncovered through which epilepsy may influence the function of this complex neuroendocrine system [16]. A potential role for the epileptic substrate has been suggested by the finding that among women with unilateral epileptic foci, PCOS is associated with left temporal and right non-temporo-limbic foci whereas hypothalamic amenorrhea has been found to be more common with right temporal lobe epilepsy [12,27] and by the finding that untreated women with primary generalized epilepsy have higher pulse frequency of GnRH secretion than normal controls [28]. Increased pulse frequency or amplitude of GnRH secretion by the hypothalamus results in preferential LH versus FSH secretion by the pituitary [29], which would promote the development of PCOS.

Effect of AEDs on endogenous hormones

Some but not all studies suggest a high prevalence of reproductive endocrine disorders in young women with epilepsy irrespective of whether or not they are treated with an AED [7]. PCOS was found to be more common among untreated (30%) than treated (13%) women with epilepsy [7]. Since this early report, the relationship between the enzyme-inhibiting AED valproate and PCOS has been demonstrated [30]. A less frequent occurrence of PCOS among women treated with enzyme-inducing AEDs such as carbamazepine has also been demonstrated in an independent investigation by Hamed *et al.* [31].

The reproductive endocrine effects of valproate in women with epilepsy was not systematically studied until the early 1990s. The first report suggesting a high incidence of menstrual disorders, linked to obesity, hyperandrogenism and polycystic ovaries, in women taking valproate for epilepsy was published in 1993 [30]. Thereafter, many studies on reproductive endocrine effects of AEDs in women with epilepsy have been published [10]. The cross-sectional study from 1993 is the only study in this field that included a large hospital-based patient population. In total, 238 women participated in the study [30]. The major finding was that menstrual disorders were common among women taking valproate monotherapy for epilepsy (45%) and that they were frequently associated with polycystic ovaries and/or hyperandrogenism, which were seen in 90% (9/10) of the women on valproate monotherapy who had menstrual disorders. Polycystic ovaries and hyperandrogenism were especially common if valproate medication was started before the age of 20. Moreover, mean serum androgen levels were increased in women on valproate [30]. Later, similar findings were obtained from a three-center study conducted in three European countries (Finland, Norway, Netherlands): menstrual disorders were reported by 59% of women on valproate compared with

12% of carbamazepine-treated women and 15% of control women. Hyperandrogenism and/or polycystic ovaries were detected in 70% of valproate-treated women compared with 20% of carbamazepine-treated women and 19% of control women. Moreover, a short-term (3 months) prospective study in newly diagnosed women starting treatment with valproate suggested that an increase in serum testosterone and androstenedione levels can be seen in approximately half of the women within 3 months after starting valproate [30].

Changes in serum androgen levels have been detected before and during pubertal development in 41 girls (8–18 years old) taking valproate for epilepsy compared with 54 healthy control girls [32]. The mean serum testosterone levels and free androgen indices were high in all pubertal phases in girls on valproate. Moreover, elevated serum testosterone levels were found in 38% of the prepubertal, 36% of the pubertal, and 57% of the postpubertal girls, whereas hyperandrogenism was seen in only 8% of the pubertal and in none of the prepubertal or postpubertal control girls [32]. A 5-year follow-up of these girls was reported later [33]. Of the girls/women who were on valproate during the follow-up study, 60% had PCOS compared with 25% of girls/women taking other AEDs, 5.5% of girls whose medication had been discontinued, and 8.3% of control subjects. Interestingly, of the 15 girls who had hyperandrogenism while on valproate during pubertal development, 71.4% (5/7) of the girls still on valproate at the time of follow-up had PCOS compared with 25% (1/4) of the girls/women who had been switched to other medication and none of four girls whose medication had been discontinued.

Four other studies have also addressed the issue of reproductive endocrine function in women with epilepsy. Luef *et al.* [34] reported a similar frequency of menstrual disorders and polycystic ovaries in women taking either carbamazepine or valproate for epilepsy. Morrell *et al.* [19] studied predictors of ovulatory failure in 94 women with epilepsy. Of women using valproate currently or within the preceding 3 years, 38.1% had experienced at least one anovulatory cycle in contrast to 10.7% of women not using valproate within the preceding 3 years. Moreover, women with idiopathic generalized epilepsy receiving valproate were at highest risk for anovulatory cycles, polycystic-appearing ovaries, elevated body mass index, and hyperandrogenism. Another study by Morrell *et al.* [35] reported higher serum testosterone levels in women taking valproate for epilepsy than in women taking lamotrigine. Finally, a study by Betts *et al.* [36] found a 30% prevalence of PCOS in women only ever treated with valproate as compared with 6% in women only ever treated with either carbamazepine or lamotrigine and 14% among healthy control women.

It seems that obesity and related hyperinsulinemia may exacerbate the valproate-related reproductive endocrine disorders in women with epilepsy.

It seems likely that valproate has a direct effect on ovarian androgen production, or as an enzyme inhibitor it may inhibit the metabolism of sex steroids and thereby lead to increased serum androgen levels.

The likelihood of developing components of PCOS with valproate treatment appears to depend on the age at which valproate is introduced. In a prospective study comparing the endocrine effects of valproate and lamotrigine in women randomized to either treatment, those beginning treatment with valproate at under 26 years of age were at highest risk for developing components of PCOS whereas those women beginning treatment with valproate at age 26 years or older had no higher risk than women with epilepsy receiving lamotrigine. In addition, the women who started valproate at the younger age had a prominent increase in serum testosterone levels [37]. This study clearly demonstrates the adverse endocrine effect of valproate on reproductive functioning as well as reproductive development.

Replacement of valproate with lamotrigine resulted in normalization of endocrine function during a 1-year follow-up in women with a previously identified reproductive endocrine disorder likely related to valproate medication. This suggests that lamotrigine therapy is not associated with changes in body weight or in endocrine and metabolic functions in women with epilepsy [10]. The reproductive endocrine effects of other new AEDs (e.g., felbamate, gabapentin, levetiracetam, pregabalin, tiagabine, topiramate, vigabatrin) have not been systematically studied in women with epilepsy [10].

Several studies have suggested that the reproductive endocrine effects of AEDs may be reversible if the medication is discontinued. In a prospective study, replacement of valproate with lamotrigine resulted in normalization of endocrine function during a 1-year follow-up in 12 women with a previously identified endocrine disorder (PCOS or hyperandrogenism or both) likely to be related to valproate medication. Serum insulin and testosterone levels returned to normal 2 months after valproate was discontinued, and the levels remained normal thereafter [9,10].

Implications for management

It is well established that most of the old AEDs (enzyme-inducing and enzyme-inhibiting drugs) have effects on reproductive function in patients with epilepsy. It is probable that epilepsy itself may modulate the regulation of reproductive endocrine function in women with epilepsy and that epilepsy may modify the effects that AEDs have on reproductive function. It is well established that AEDs with liver enzyme-inducing properties decrease the serum concentrations of bioactive sex steroids, whereas valproate increases the serum concentrations of androgens. To identify and treat reproductive disorders, women with epilepsy should be asked routinely about commonly occurring problems such as weight gain, abnormal menstrual cycle length or irregularity, mid-cycle spotting, hirsutism, or acne. Suspicion of AED-induced PCOS may warrant an endocrine screen, including LH, testosterone and prolactin levels, and ovarian ultrasound.

It is important to acknowledge that the reproductive effects of AEDs may be different depending on the age. Young women with epilepsy seem to be especially vulnerable to the effects of valproate on ovarian function. The endocrine effects of the new AEDs have not been widely studied. However, it seems they may offer an alternative if reproductive endocrine problems emerge during treatment with the older AEDs. It is encouraging to note that most of the reproductive effects of the AEDs appear to be reversible if the medication is discontinued before adulthood. Changing to an alternative AED may be considered.

Review of the case: A young woman of childbearing age, treated with topiramate for temporal lobe epilepsy, suffered from menstrual cycle disturbances. She reported abnormal variation in cycle intervals and particularly strong menstrual cycles and anovulatory cycles were diagnosed as well. She did not become pregnant within 3 years after withdrawal from her oral contraceptive pill.

She seemed to be free of epileptic seizures because she reported no tonic–clonic seizures or seizures with loss of awareness for more than 10 years. However, she misinterpreted epigastric auras as panic attacks and she still had complex partial seizures, only demonstrated at the epilepsy video monitoring unit. Topiramate was switched to levetiracetam and she reported improvement of menstrual cycle disorders weeks later and no prior observed "panic attacks" (auras). She is free of seizures.

Topiramate is not an enzyme-inducing or enzyme-inhibiting drug and is not known to have any influence on the menstrual cycle. Topiramate is known for reducing body weight, and higher body mass index is associated with a higher risk for development of PCOS including menstrual cycle disorders. Theoretically, topiramate could be a drug preventing menstrual cycle disturbances in overweight women with epilepsy.

Epilepsy can be associated with reproductive endocrine disorders. In women these include PCOS, isolated components of this syndrome such as polycystic ovaries or hyperandrogenemia, menstrual cycle disturbances, hypothalamic amenorrhea, or functional hyperprolactinemia. The most likely explanation for endocrine disorders related to epilepsy is a direct influence on the endocrine control centers in the brain (hypothalamic–pituitary axis).

Therefore, regular monitoring of reproductive function at visits, including questioning about menstrual disorders, fertility, weight, hirsutism, and galactorrhea, are recommended. Single abnormal laboratory or imaging findings without symptoms may not constitute a clinically relevant endocrine disorder. However, patients with these kinds of abnormalities should be monitored in order to detect the possible development of a symptomatic disorder associated with, for example, menstrual disorders or fertility problems. If a reproductive endocrine disorder is subsequently found, AEDs should be reviewed in terms of their indication for the particular seizure type and their tolerability vis-à-vis their potential for contributing to the endocrine problem as well to reanalyze for possible seizures.

Key summary points

- It is well established that AEDs with liver enzyme-inducing properties decrease the serum concentrations of bioactive sex steroids, whereas valproate increases the serum concentrations of androgens.

- It is probable that epilepsy itself may modulate the regulation of reproductive endocrine function in women with epilepsy and that epilepsy may modify the effects that AEDs have on reproductive function.

- To identify and treat reproductive disorders, women with epilepsy should be asked routinely about commonly occurring problems such as weight gain, abnormal menstrual cycle length or irregularity, mid-cycle spotting, hirsutism, or acne.

- Suspicion of AED-induced PCOS may warrant an endocrine screen, including LH, testosterone and prolactin levels, and ovarian ultrasound.

- The reproductive effects of AEDs may be different depending on the age; young women with epilepsy seem to be especially vulnerable to the effects of valproate on ovarian function.

- The reproductive effects of AEDs appear to be reversible and if adverse reproductive endocrine effects are present, changing to an alternative AED should be considered.

References

1 Webber MP, Hauser WA, Ottman R, Annegers JF. Fertility in persons with epilepsy: 1935–1974. *Epilepsia* 1986;27:746–752.

2 Wallace H, Shorvon S, Tallis R. Age-specific incidence and prevalence rates of treated epilepsy in an unselected population of 2,052,922 and age-specific fertility rates of women with epilepsy. *Lancet* 1998;352:1970–1973.

3 Dansky LV, Andermann E, Andermann F. Marriage and fertility in epileptic patients. *Epilepsia* 1980;21:261–271.

4 Schupf N, Ottman R. Reproduction among individuals with idiopathic/cryptogenic epilepsy: risk factors for reduced fertility inmarriage. *Epilepsia* 1996;37:833–840.

5 Tauboll E, Luef G. Gender issues in epilepsy: the science of why it is special. *Seizure* 2008;17:99–100.

6 Herzog AG. A hypothesis to integrate partial seizures of temporal lobe origin and reproductive disorders. *Epilepsy Res* 1989;3:151–159.

7 Herzog AG, Seibel MM, Schomer DL, Vaitukaitis JL, Geschwind N. Reproductive endocrine disorders in women with partial seizures of temporal lobe origin. *Arch Neurol* 1986;43:341–346.

8 Herzog AG, Seibel MM, Schomer DL, Vaitukaitis JL, Geschwind N. Reproductive endocrine disorders in men with partial seizures of temporal lobe origin. *Arch Neurol* 1986;43:347–350.

9 Margraf JW, Dreifuss FE. Amenorrhea following initiation of therapy with valproic acid. [Abstract] *Neurology* 1981;31(Suppl):159.

10 Isojärvi J. Disorders of reproduction in patients with epilepsy: antiepileptic drug related mechanisms. *Seizure* 2008;17:111–119.

11 Luef G, Rauchenzauner M. Epilepsy and hormones: a critical review. *Epilepsy Behav* 2009;15:73–77.

12 Herzog AG. A relationship between particular reproductive endocrine disorders and the laterality of epileptiform discharges in women with epilepsy. *Neurology* 1993;43:1907–1910.

13 Luef G. Hormonal alterations following seizures. *Epilepsy Behav* 2010;19:131–133.

14 Herzog AG, Coleman AE, Jacobs AR *et al*. Interictal EEG discharges, reproductive hormones and menstrual disorders in epilepsy. *Ann Neurol* 2003;54:625–37.

15 Herzog AG, Friedman MN. Menstrual cycle interval and ovulation in women with localization-related epilepsy. *Neurology* 2002;57:2133–2135.

16 Herzog AG. Disorders of reproduction in patients with epilepsy: primary neurological mechanisms. *Seizure* 2008;17:101–110.

17 Herzog AG, Klein P, Ransil BJ. Three patterns of catamenial epilepsy. *Epilepsia* 1997;38:1082–1088.

18 Cummings LN, Morrell MJ, Giudice L. Ovulatory function in epilepsy. *Epilepsia* 1995;36:353–357.

19 Morrell MJ, Giudice L, Flynn KL *et al*. Predictors of ovulatory failure in women with epilepsy. *Ann Neurol* 2002;52:704–711.

20 Harden CL, Koppel BS, Herzog AG, Nikolov BG, Hauser WA. Seizure frequency is associated with age of menopause in women with epilepsy. *Neurology* 2003;61:451–455.

21 Lofgren E, Mikkonen K, Tolonen U *et al*. Reproductive endocrine function in women with epilepsy: the role of epilepsy type and medication. *Epilepsy Behav* 2007;10:77–83.

22 Schupf N, Ottman R. Likelihood of pregnancy in individuals with idiopathic/cryptogenic epilepsy: social and biologic influences. *Epilepsia* 1994;35:750–756.

23 Herzog AG. Reproductive endocrine regulation in men with epilepsy: effects on reproductive function and neuronal excitability. *Ann Neurol* 2002;51:539–542.

24 Herzog AG, Schachter SC. On the association between valproate and polycystic ovary syndrome. *Epilepsia* 2001:42:311–315.

25 Eagleson CA, Gingrich MB, Pastor CL *et al*. Polycystic ovarian syndrome: evidence that flutamide restores sensitivity of the gonadotropin-releasing hormone pulse generator to inhibition by estradiol and progesterone. *J Clin Endocrinol Metab* 2000;85:4047–4052.

26 Spratt DI, Finkelstein JS, Butler JP, Badger TM, Crowley WF Jr. Effects of increasing the frequency of low doses of gonadotropin releasing hormone (GnRH) on gonadotropin secretion in GnRH-deficient men. *J Clin Endocrinol Metab* 1987;64:1179.

27 Kalinin VV, Zheleznova EV. Chronology and evolution of temporal lobe epilepsy and endocrine reproductive function in females. Relationships with foci laterality and catameniality. *Epilepsy Behav* 2007;11:185–191.

28 Bilo L, Meo R, Valentino R, Buscaino GA, Striano S, Nappi C. Abnormal patterns of luteinizing hormone pulsatility in women with epilepsy. *Fertil Steril* 1991;55: 705–711.

29 Knobil E. The neuroendocrine control of the menstrual cycle. *Recent Prog Horm Res* 1980;36:53–80.

30 Isojärvi JI, Laatikainen TJ, Pakarinen AJ, Juntunen KT, Myllylä VV. Polycystic ovaries and hyperandrogenism in women taking valproate for epilepsy. *N Engl J Med* 1993;329:1383–1388.

31 Hamed SA, Hamed EA, Shokry M, Omar H, Abdellah MM. The reproductive conditions and lipid profile in females with epilepsy. *Acta Neurol Scand* 2007;115:12–22.

32 Vainionpää LK, Rättyä J, Knip M *et al*. Valproate-induced hyperandrogenism during pubertal maturation in girls with epilepsy. *Ann Neurol* 1999;45:444–450.

33 Mikkonen K, Vainionpää LK, Pakarinen AJ *et al*. Long-term reproductive endocrine health in young women with epilepsy during puberty. *Neurology* 2004;62:445–450.

34 Luef G, Abraham I, Haslinger M *et al*. Polycystic ovaries, obesity and insulin resistance in women with epilepsy. A comparative study of carbamazepine and valproic acid in 105 women. *J Neurol* 2002;249:835–841.

35 Morrell M, Bhatt M, Ozkara C *et al*. Higher incidence of symptoms of polycystic ovary syndrome in women with epilepsy treated with valproate versus lamotrigine. *Neurology* 2005;64(Suppl 1):428.

36 Betts T, Yarrow H, Dutton N, Greenhill L, Rolfe T. A study of anticonvulsant medication on ovarian function in a group of women with epilepsy who have only ever taken one anticonvulsant compared with a group of women without epilepsy. *Seizure* 2003;12:323–329.

37 Morrell MJ, Hayes FJ, Sluss PM *et al*. Hyperandrogenism, ovulatory dysfunction, and polycystic ovary syndrome with valproate versus lamotrigine. *Ann Neurol* 2008;64.200–211.

CHAPTER 6

Contraception and Epilepsy

Anne R. Davis and Kathleen M. Morrell

Department of Obstetrics and Gynecology, Columbia University Medical Center, New York, USA

Case history: *J.R. is a 23-year-old woman who presents to your office to discuss birth control. Her medical history includes well-controlled partial epilepsy currently treated by monotherapy with 600 mg daily carbamazepine (CBZ). She reports being told by doctors in the past that she would have problems using hormonal birth control because of her antiepileptic medications. She also suffers from heavy menstrual bleeding, and asks about treatment options for this as well. She is sexually active, has a history of one voluntary abortion at age 19, and uses male condoms for birth control now. She plans pregnancy in about 5 years.*

Background and important detail

Even women who choose to bear several children must use contraceptives for roughly three decades [1]. There is a variety of contraceptive methods available, the most effective methods including male and female sterilization, intrauterine devices (IUDs), and the contraceptive implant (etonogestrel implant) (Table 6.1). These require little or no effort on the part of the user, and typically have a failure rate of about one pregnancy per 100 women per year. Unlike sterilization, baseline fertility returns immediately after removal of an IUD or the implant. Other very effective hormonal methods of contraception include the daily oral contraceptive pill (OC), weekly transdermal patch, monthly vaginal ring (ethinyl estradiol and etonogestrel vaginal ring) and 3-month medroxyprogester-one injection. These are the most commonly used forms in the USA, with OCs being the most frequently used by far [2]. These short-term methods have lower efficacy rates of about 6–10 pregnancies per 100 women per year; these pregnancies result from variable adherence and access over time. The least effective methods include male and female condoms, diaphragm, sponge, spermicides, withdrawal, and fertility awareness methods. More than 12 pregnancies per 100 women per year can occur among users who rely on these less-effective methods [3].

Table 6.1 Contraceptives available in the USA.

Method	Efficacy*	Reversibility	Effect on bleeding	Duration of use	Ovulation inhibition?
Oral contraceptive pill	88–94%	Immediate	Decreased, regular	Daily	Yes
Transdermal patch	88–94%	Immediate	Decreased, regular	Weekly	Yes
Vaginal ring	88–94%	Immediate	Decreased, regular	Monthly	Yes
Depot medroxyprogesterone acetate (DMPA)	88–94%	Delayed†	Initially irregular, amenorrhea likely with continuation	Every 3 months	Yes
Subdermal implant	>99%	Immediate	Decreased, irregular	3 years	Yes
Levonorgestrel IUD	>99%	Immediate	Decreased, initially irregular	5 years	Sometimes
Copper IUD	>99%	Immediate	Sometimes increased, regular	10 years	No

*With typical use, per year assuming no drug interactions present.
†Median return to ovulation >6 months from time of last injection.

Guidelines recommend highly effective contraception for women with epilepsy to prevent exposure to teratogenic antiepileptic drugs (AEDs) and to optimize seizure control prior to pregnancy [4]. However, the contraceptive behaviors of women with epilepsy have received little study. One cross-sectional questionnaire study indicated that contraception for women with epilepsy remains problematic, despite published guidelines. In this sample of 145 reproductive-age women with epilepsy at an urban medical center, only 53% of those at risk of unplanned pregnancy reported current use of a highly effective method and 50% of all their reported pregnancies were unplanned [5].

Hormonal contraceptive methods

Hormonal contraception is safe, well tolerated, and commonly used among healthy women. Current available options include progestin-only forms and methods that combine an estrogen and a progestin. Progestin-only methods are available in the form of pills, an injectable, an implant, and an IUD, specifically the levonorgestrel-releasing intrauterine system. The injectable contains medroxyprogesterone acetate given every 3 months. The 3-year implant and the 5-year IUD release etonogestrel or levonorgestrel, respectively, after placement.

Progestin-only methods are particularly safe; their use does not increase the risk of thrombosis associated with estrogen-containing methods.

All progestin-only methods thicken cervical mucus and prevent passage of sperm. Depot medroxyprogesterone acetate (DMPA) and the implant also inhibit ovulation. Ovulation occurs erratically on progestin-only pills and the progestin IUD.

The combined methods include OCs, the transdermal patch, and the vaginal ring. All three inhibit ovulation centrally. These methods combine one of two estrogen formulations (ethinyl estradiol or estradiol valerate) with one of various different progestins. OC preparations vary by the number of hormone-free days: (i) four hormone-free days per month, (ii) one hormone-free week per month, (iii) four hormone-free weeks per year, or (iv) continuous usage without any hormone-free days. Overall, the expected noncontraceptive benefits for all combined hormonal methods include improved dysmenorrhea and acne, decreased menstrual bleeding, and reduced risk of endometrial and ovarian cancer [6].

Pharmacokinetic interactions between contraceptive hormones and AEDs

Women with epilepsy face particular challenges that make use of hormonal contraception complex, for both themselves and their health-care providers. Most women with epilepsy are maintained on at least one AED for years. Some AEDs induce the hepatic cytochrome P450 enzyme system (enzyme-inducing AEDs), which augments the metabolism of contraceptive steroids. Inducers include drugs such as oxcarbazepine, CBZ, primidone, phenytoin, phenobarbital, felbamate and, to a lesser extent, topiramate, clobazam, and lamotrigine (Table 6.2).

Multiple published pharmacokinetic studies demonstrate that enzyme induction via AED exposure lowers serum levels of orally administered contraceptive steroids. Most inducers decrease estrogen and progestins. Two exceptions are topiramate and lamotrigine. Topiramate decreases ethinyl estradiol, but not progestin. This occurs in a dose-related manner: doses of topiramate of up to 200 mg/day are associated with an estradiol decrease in area under the concentration curve (AUC) of up to 18%, and doses of 400–800 mg/day are associated with an estradiol AUC decrease of 22–30% [7,8]. Lamotrigine decreases progestin, modestly by up to 20%, but not the ethinyl estradiol component [9].

Pharmacokinetic studies cannot determine the impact of the drug interaction on risk of pregnancy. However, these pharmacokinetic changes likely do contribute to an increased risk of contraceptive failure when women take AEDs and OCs together. One report showed a clearly increased

Table 6.2 Antiepileptic drugs.

Enzyme-inducing antiepileptic drugs
Phenobarbital
Primidone
Phenytoin
Carbamazepine
Oxcarbazepine
Felbamate
Topiramate* (dose dependent)
Lamotrigine[†]
Clobazam

Nonenzyme-inducing antiepileptic drugs
Ethosuximide
Clonazepam
Valproic acid
Vigabatrin
Gabapentin
Levetiracetam
Pregabalin
Lacosamide
Ezogabine (INN retigabine)

---

*Decreases ethinyl estradiol, but no change in progestin level.
[†]Lamotrigine decreases progestin, no change in ethinyl estradiol level.

pregnancy rate in the setting of women taking OCs and AEDs compared with women taking OCs alone (relative risk 25, 95% confidence interval 5–73) [10]. Lack of suppression of ovulation due to a known pharmacokinetic interaction has been shown in a recent study. This investigation examined pharmacokinetic changes with an enzyme-inducing AED and the physiologic indicators of pregnancy risk during OC use. In this cross-over study of healthy women ($N=10$), administration of CBZ 600 mg lowered OC hormone levels (20 μg ethinyl estradiol with 150 mg levonorgestrel) compared to the same OC coadministered with a placebo [11]. These lower levels resulted in ovulation and breakthrough bleeding during CBZ exposure compared with placebo. These two clinical pharmacodynamic changes with concomitant low-dose OCs and CBZ resulted in an unacceptably increased risk of pregnancy. Indeed, case reports confirm pregnancies during CBZ and OC use, even with higher-dose OCs [12,13]. Results from this study may not be generalizable to other enzyme-inducing AEDs since the degree of enzyme induction is variable.

Drug interactions during OC and AED coadministration can also affect safety by adversely impacting seizure control. This type of interaction is best understood for lamotrigine. The concentration of lamotrigine decreases when taken in combination with OCs [14,15] probably related to ethinyl estradiol-induced glucuronidation [16]. Additionally, recent data also raise the possibility that OCs affect levels of valproic acid, another commonly used AED [15]. Such interactions necessitate adjustment of AED dosing based on cyclic changes in OC dose, creating a risk for breakthrough seizures and increasing the complexity of care for women with epilepsy.

For women treated with glucuronidated AEDs, progestin-only methods obviate estrogen-mediated decreases in AED levels. Therefore, the World Health Organization Expert Working Group determined that for women using lamotrigine monotherapy, it is appropriate to consider progestogen-only contraceptives, i.e., pills, DMPA, norethisterone enanthate (another depot injectable progestin), the levonorgestrel or etonogestrel implant, or the levonorgestrel-releasing intrauterine system [17]. Case reports document pregnancies during concomitant use of phenobarbital or phenytoin with the levonorgestrel implant [18–20] and CBZ with the etonogestrel implant [21]; however, these are strong inducers.

Hormone–AED interactions have not been studied for other nonoral combined contraceptive methods such as the hormonal ring or patch. As these are also metabolized by the cytochrome P450 system in the liver, we would expect similar effects.

Hormonal contraception and seizure control

The safety of combined hormonal contraception in terms of seizure control, independent of AED-mediated effects, remains unknown. In human and animal models, estrogen has proconvulsant properties whereas progesterone, and in particular its active metabolite allopregnanolone, have anticonvulsant properties [22]. Hormonal modulation of the seizure threshold is particularly important for women with catamenial epilepsy. Despite known hormonal influences on seizures and OC popularity, no study has examined the impact of OCs on seizure frequency. However, one large epidemiologic study demonstrated no increased risk in the diagnosis of epilepsy during use of OCs [23].

The DMPA injection, given every 3 months, administers higher levels of progestin than the implant. One small study ($N=19$) from 1984 prospectively examined the effect of oral and/or intramuscular medroxyprogesterone acetate (as a 3-month injection) on seizures in women with refractory partial epilepsy. This study reported a reduction in seizure frequency for half of the patients within 1 year of follow-up. However, the results are difficult to interpret: the study was small, had no control group, and patients were given variable doses of oral and intramuscular medroxyprogesterone acetate. In animal models, some data suggest certain progestins are preferable for their anticonvulsant effects, but there are no data in humans suggesting that one type of contraceptive progestin is superior to another with regard to seizure control [24]. Of all the contraceptive methods available, DMPA is the only one proven to cause a decrease in bone mineral density (BMD) [25,26]. Studies suggest that persons with epilepsy treated with some AEDs have an increased risk of fracture, low BMD, and abnormalities in bone metabolism. Given the potential of a compounded effect on BMD with concurrent AED use, the use of DMPA as a contraceptive method in women with epilepsy should be individualized (see Chapter 19).

Intrauterine contraception

Intrauterine contraception provides a simple, low-maintenance, "forgettable" method for women managing a chronic medical condition. High efficacy provides security; women can avoid AED-related teratogenicity in an unplanned pregnancy. The copper IUD is a nonhormonal form that is approved for 10 years of use, while the progestin-only levonorgestrel IUD lasts for 5 years. Both IUDs are placed in the office by a clinician and are appropriate for use in nulliparous women [27]. The main mechanism of action for hormonal intrauterine contraception is local via thickening of cervical mucus. This local effect is probably less susceptible to the hepatic-mediated drug interactions which decrease the effectiveness of centrally acting oral contraception. After an initial rise, progestin released by this IUD rapidly falls to a level too low to inhibit ovulation. One reassuring prospective questionnaire-based study demonstrated a pregnancy rate of 1.1 per 100 women-years for 56 women using the levonorgestrel intrauterine system (LNG-IUS) with enzyme-inducing AEDs, a rate slightly higher than expected but still very low compared with other contraceptive methods [28]. Intrauterine contraception obviates estrogen-mediated decrease in AED levels and associated breakthrough seizures, and the hypothetical negative effects of estrogen itself on seizure threshold.

Dual benefit of pregnancy prevention and decreased menstrual bleeding

Several methods of contraception offer the dual benefit of pregnancy prevention and decreased menstrual bleeding. OCs reduce menstrual blood loss when used cyclically or in extended cycle or continuous regimens [29,30]. One OC containing estradiol valerate has been shown in studies to have fewer days of bleeding overall compared with other OCs containing ethinyl estradiol [31,32]. This OC has been studied with the most rigorous methodology, but it has not been compared with other OCs. DMPA and the implant initially cause menstrual irregularity, but both result in decreased bleeding over time [33–35]. Half of DMPA users experience amenorrhea after 1 year and up to 80% will after 5 years. Menstrual blood loss is reduced 90% for users of the levonorgestrel IUD and 20% of its users will experience amenorrhea [36–39]. In 2009, the US Food and Drug Administration approved the levonorgestrel IUD for treatment of heavy menstrual bleeding [40]. The copper IUD would be a specific method to avoid in patients like J.R. who experience heavy menses; more than half of women experience increased bleeding during use of the copper IUD [41,42].

Implications for management

In addressing the needs of our case patient J.R., our first consideration would be efficacy in preventing pregnancy while preserving future fertility. Since J.R. takes CBZ, the known, potent enzyme-inducing properties of this AED will decrease contraceptive efficacy of OCs, and probably the patch and the ring as well. J.R. experiences heavy menstrual bleeding. Some contraceptive methods have the dual purposes of preventing pregnancy and reducing menstrual blood loss. Ideally, her method should provide dual benefits. The next concern would be how any new contraceptive method may affect her seizures. Other than the concerns with lamotrigine levels being lowered with concurrent OC use, there is minimal direct evidence regarding how, and if, different contraceptive methods impact seizure frequency and/or severity. J.R. is not seeking pregnancy soon; however, any teratogenic effect of her current AED regimen should be addressed when discussing contraception.

Review of the case: In discussion with patient J.R., we would not recommend combined hormonal methods (OC, patch or ring), progestin-only pills or implants, or the copper IUD for her contraceptive needs. Combined hormonal methods would likely improve J.R.'s heavy menstrual bleeding, but documented decreased OC efficacy and breakthrough bleeding with concomitant CBZ is concerning for all similarly acting forms. Pregnancies reported in women using the progestin-only implants on potent enzyme-inducing AEDs, such as CBZ, make this a poor contraceptive choice. The copper IUD would be a very effective contraceptive and obviates any drug interactions, but her heavy menstrual bleeding would not improve and may worsen.

DMPA may fulfill all of J.R.'s needs. This method is highly effective, does not require daily adherence, and with continued use would dramatically decrease menstrual bleeding. The effect of CBZ on DMPA pharmacokinetics is unknown. The high doses achieved with this injectable are reassuring, even if P450 enzyme induction impacts metabolism of DMPA. However, the potential for a further decrease in BMD with DMPA use is concerning.

The levonorgestrel intrauterine system may be an ideal method. Like DMPA, this method is highly effective, does not require daily adherence, and with continued use would help her heavy menstrual bleeding. This method is safe in nulliparous women like J.R. When she desires pregnancy, unlike DMPA, she could expect a rapid return to fertility after removal. Normal ovulation may take up to 1 year to return after discontinuing use of DMPA [43]. The contraceptive efficacy of the levonorgestrel IUD relies on its local intrauterine effects, so hepatic-mediated drug interactions probably do not affect efficacy in a clinically important way.

 Key summary points

- Women with epilepsy need highly effective contraception to prevent pregnancy, but also to prevent exposure to teratogenic AEDs and to allow them to optimize seizure control prior to pregnancy.

- Some AEDs induce the hepatic cytochrome P450 system, which can lower serum levels of contraceptive steroids; potent inducers increase pregnancy risk for OCs and probably vaginal ring and patch.

- The serum concentration of lamotrigine decreases when taken in combination with OCs containing ethinyl estradiol.

- Progesterone-only hormonal contraceptives may be considered for women taking lamotrigine monotherapy.

- The safety of estrogen-containing hormonal contraception in terms of seizure control for women with epilepsy remains unclear.

- Pregnancies have been reported in women using a progestin-only subdermal implant with concurrent use of potent enzyme-inducing AEDs.

- Intrauterine contraception is safe in nulliparous women. The progestin-only IUD decreases menstrual bleeding.

- Return to baseline fertility can take up to 1 year after DMPA administration.

- Many contraceptive methods have the dual benefits of preventing pregnancy and improving menstrual irregularities.

References

1 Guttmacher Institute. Facts on contraceptive use in the United States. Available at www.guttmacher.org/pubs/fb_contr_use.pdf, accessed December 2, 2011.
2 Mosher WD, Jones J. Use of contraception in the United States: 1982–2008. *Vital Health Stat 23* 2010;(29):1–44.

3 Trussell J, Guthrie KA. Choosing a contraceptive: efficacy, safety and personal considerations. In: Kowal D (ed.) *Contraceptive Technology, 20th* revised edn. New York: Ardent Media, Inc., 2011: 45–74.

4 Practice Parameter. Management issues for women with epilepsy (summary statement). Report of the Quality Standards Subcommittee of the American Academy of Neurology. *Neurology* 1998;51:944–948.

5 Davis AR, Pack AM, Kritzer J, Yoon A, Camus A. Reproductive history, sexual behavior and use of contraception in women with epilepsy. *Contraception* 2008;77:405–409.

6 Nelson AL, Cwiak C. Combined oral contraceptives (COCs). In: Kowal D (ed.) *Contraceptive Technology, 20th* revised edn. New York: Ardent Media, Inc., 2011: 249–341.

7 Doose DR, Wang S, Padmanabhan M, Schwabe S, Jacobs D, Bialer M. Effect of topiramate or CBZ on the pharmacokinetics of an oral contraceptive containing norethindrone and ethinyl estradiol in healthy obese and nonobese female subjects. *Epilepsia* 2003;44:540–549.

8 Rosenfeld WE, Doose DR, Walker SA, Nayak RK. Effect of topiramate on the pharmacokinetics of an oral contraceptive containing norethindrone and ethinyl estradiol in patients with epilepsy. *Epilepsia* 1997;38:317–323.

9 Sidhu J, Job S, Singh S, Philipson R. The pharmacokinetic and pharmacodynamic consequences of the co-administration of lamotrigine and a combined oral contraceptive in health female subjects. *Br J Clin Pharmacol* 2005;61:191–199.

10 Coulam CB, Annegers JF. Do anticonvulsants reduce the efficacy of oral contraceptives? *Epilepsia* 1979;20:519–525.

11 Davis AR, Westhoff CL, Stanczyk FZ. Carbamazepine coadministration with an oral contraceptive: effects on steroid pharmacokinetics, ovulation, and bleeding. *Epilepsia* 2011;52:243–247.

12 Back DJ, Grimmer SF, Orme ML, Proudlove C, Mann RD, Breckenridge AM. Evaluation of Committee on Safety of Medicines yellow card reports on oral contraceptive-drug interactions with anti-convulsants and antibiotics. *Br J Clin Pharmacol* 1988;25:527–532.

13 Kenyon IE. Unplanned pregnancy in an epileptic. *Br Med J* 1972;1:686–687.

14 Burakgazi E, Harden C, Kelly JJ. Contraception for women with epilepsy. *Rev Neurol Dis* 2009;6:E62–E67.

15 Herzog AG, Blum AS, Farina EL *et al.* Valproate and lamotrigine level variation with menstrual cycle phase and oral contraceptive use. *Neurology* 2009;72:911–914.

16 Reimers A, Helde G, Brodtkorb E. Ethinyl estradiol, not progestogens, reduces lamotrigine serum concentrations. *Epilepsia* 2005;46:1414–1417.

17 Gaffield ME, Culwell KR, Lee CR. The use of hormonal contraception among women taking anticonvulsant therapy. *Contraception* 2011;83:16–29.

18 Shane-McWhorter L, Cerveny JD, MacFarlane LL, Osborn C. Enhanced metabolism of levonorgestrel during phenobarbital treatment and resultant pregnancy. *Pharmacotherapy* 1998;18:1360–1364.

19 Odlind V, Olsson SE. Enhanced metabolism of levonorgestrel during phenytoin treatment in a woman with Norplant implants. *Contraception* 1986;33:257–261.

20 Haukkamaa M. Contraception by Norplant subdermal capsules is not reliable in epileptic patients on anticonvulsant treatment. *Contraception* 1986;33:559–565.

21 Schindlbeck C, Janni W, Friese K. Failure of Implanon contraception in a patient taking carbamazepin for epilepsia. *Arch Gynecol Obstet* 2006;273:255–256.

22 Reddy DS, Rogawski MA. Neurosteroid replacement therapy for catamenial epilepsy. *Neurotherapeutics* 2009;6:392–401.

23 Vessey M, Painter R, Yeates D. Oral contraception and epilepsy: findings in a large cohort study. *Contraception* 2002;66:77–79.

24 Frye CA. Hormonal influences on seizures: basic neurobiology. In: Gidal BE, Harden CL (eds) *Epilepsy in Women: The Scientific Basics for Clinical Management.* New York: Elsevier, 2008: 27–77.

25 Clark MK, Sowers M, Levy B, Nichols S. Bone mineral density loss and recovery during 48 months in first-time users of depot medroxyprogesterone acetate. *Fertil Steril* 2006;86:1466–1474.

26 Cundy T, Cornish J, Roberts H, Elder H, Reid I. Spinal bone density in women using depot medroxyprogesterone acetate contraception. *Obstet Gynecol* 1998;92:569–573.

27 American College of Obstetricians and Gynecologists. *Long-Acting Reversible Contraception: Implants and Intrauterine Devices.* ACOG Practice Bulletin No. 121. Washington, DC: ACOG, 2011.

28 Bounds W, Guillebaud J. Observational series on women using the contraceptive Mirena concurrently with anti-epileptic and other enzyme-inducing drugs. *J Fam Plann Reprod Health Care* 2002;28:78–80.

29 Farquhar C, Brown J. Oral contraceptive pill for heavy menstrual bleeding. *Cochrane Database Syst Rev* 2009;(4):CD000154.

30 Miller L, Notter KM. Menstrual reduction with extended use of combination oral contraceptive pills: randomized controlled trial. *Obstet Gynecol* 2001;98:771–778.

31 Ahrendt H, Makalova D, Parke S, Mellinger U, Mansour D. Bleeding pattern and cycle control with an estradiol-based oral contraceptive: a seven-cycle, randomized comparative trial of estradiol valerate/dienogest and ethinyl estradiol/levonorgestrel. *Contraception* 2009;80:436–444.

32 Jensen JT, Parke S, Mellinger Q, Machlitt A, Fraser IS. Effective treatment of heavy menstrual bleeding with estradiol valerate and dienogest: a randomized controlled trial. *Obstet Gynecol* 2011;117:777–787.

33 Schwialle PC, Assenzo JR. Contraceptive use: efficacy study utilizing medroxyprogesterone acetate administered as an intramuscular injection once every 90 days. *Fertil Steril* 1973;24:331–339.

34 Belsey EM. Vaginal bleeding patterns among women using one natural and eight hormonal methods of contraception. *Contraception* 1988;38:181–206.

35 Power J, French R, Cowan F. Subdermal implantable contraceptives versus other forms of reversible contraceptives or other implants as effective methods for preventing pregnancy. *Cochrane Database Syst Rev* 2007;(3):CD001326.

36 Istre O, Trolle B. Treatment of menorrhagia with the levonorgestrel intrauterine system versus endometrial resection. *Fertil Steril* 2001;76:304–309.

37 Barrington JW, Bowen-Simpkins P. The levonorgestrel intrauterine system in the management of menorrhagia. *Br J Obstet Gynaecol* 1997;104:614–616.

38 Tang GWK, Lo SST. Levonorgestrel intrauterine device in the treatment of menorrhagia in Chinese women: efficacy versus acceptability. *Contraception* 1995;51:231–235.

39 Andersson JK, Rybo G. Levonorgestrel-releasing intrauterine device in the treatment of menorrhagia. *Br J Obstet Gynaecol* 1990;97:690–694.

40 US Food and Drug Administration. FDA approves additional use for IUD Mirena to treat heavy menstrual bleeding in IUD users. www.fda.gov/NewsEvents/Newsroom/PressAnnouncements/ucm184747.htm, accessed December 9, 2011.

41 Sivin I, Stern J. Health during prolonged use of levonorgestrel 20 micrograms/d and the copper TCu 380Ag intrauterine contraceptive devices: a multicenter study. *Fertil Steril* 1994;61:70–77.

42 Hubacher D. Side effects from the copper IUD: do they decrease over time? *Contraception* 2009;79:356–362.

43 Paulen ME, Curtis KM. When can a woman have repeat progestogen-only injectables: depot medroxyprogesterone acetate or northisterone enantate? *Contraception* 2009;80:391–408.

CHAPTER 7

Diagnostic Challenges with Seizures in Pregnancy

Sanjeev V. Thomas

Department of Neurology, Sree Chitra Tirunal Institute for Medical Sciences and Technology, Trivandrum, Kerala, India

---

Case history: *A 19-year-old woman (gravida 1, para 1) presented with generalized seizures on the fourth postpartum day. She had preeclampsia during pregnancy but had an uneventful delivery. The baby weighed 2.8 kg and thrived well. The patient had generalized headache from the third postpartum day. The next day she had one episode of focal jerking of left leg followed by a generalized tonic–clonic seizure. Her physical examination revealed that she was afebrile and blood pressure was 130/90 mmHg; there was no lymphadenopathy or pedal edema. She was drowsy. Her optic fundi showed papilledema, there was mild weakness of left foot and neck stiffness. Magnesium sulfate 4 g was administered intravenously with 6 g intramuscularly as loading dose. She had one more seizure about 2 hours after admission. Urine proteins were present. Magnetic resonance imaging (MRI) of the brain revealed focal areas of increased T2 signal over right posterior frontal and parietal area and magnetic resonance venography demonstrated occlusion of the superior sagittal sinus with opening up of collaterals.*

Seizures in pregnancy

Acute seizure is an alarming complication during pregnancy and calls for emergency evaluation and prompt management. Epilepsy is one of the most common causes of seizures during pregnancy. More than half of women with epilepsy experience no change or an improvement in seizure control during pregnancy, probably due to the protective effect of progesterone. Seizure exacerbation is most likely during the peripartum period than other months of pregnancy [1] (see Chapter 8 for more details). Nevertheless, seizures can exacerbate during the first or last trimester. This is mainly due to the rapid changes in the ovarian hormonal profile, sleep deprivation, or emotional disturbances. In the early period of pregnancy,

---

Epilepsy in Women, First Edition. Edited by Cynthia L. Harden, Sanjeev V. Thomas and Torbjörn Tomson.

Table 7.1 Causes of seizures during pregnancy.

I	**Hemodynamic disorders**
	Eclampsia
	Posterior reversible encephalopathy syndrome
II	**Vascular**
A	*Malformations*
	Arteriovenous malformation
	Cavernoma
B	*Stroke*
	Cerebral venous thrombosis
	Postpartum cerebral angiopathy
	Antiphospholipid antibody syndrome, vasculitis
III	**Autoimmune disorders**
A	*Autoimmune encephalitis*
	N-methyl-D-aspartate receptor antibody-associated encephalitides
	Late-onset Rasmussen encephalitis
	Limbic encephalitis
B	*Autoimmune systemic disorders*
	Hashimoto encephalopathy
	Systemic lupus erythematosus
	Amniotic fluid embolism
IV	**Infections**
A	*Viral encephalitis*
	Herpes simplex, dengue, varicella, HIV
B	*Bacterial*
	Brain abscess, listeriosis
	Tuberculoma
C	*Others*
	Toxoplasmosis
	Malaria
	Neurocysticercosis
V	**Brain tumors**
VI	**Metabolic disorders**
VII	**Substance abuse**
	Alcohol
	Cocaine
	Others

excessive vomiting with difficulty in retaining medications and metabolic or hormonal changes can predispose a woman being treated for epilepsy to suffer seizures. In the second and third trimester, the blood levels of antiepileptic drugs (AEDs) may decline and thereby permit seizures. New-onset epilepsy can also start during this period. Incidence studies indicate that a substantial proportion of new-onset epilepsy begins in young adulthood, when most pregnancies occur. Hence it is possible that a woman may experience the first seizure of her epilepsy during pregnancy. Seizures during pregnancy can be due to several other causes (Table 7.1). The objective of this chapter is to briefly discuss some of the different causes and outline a strategy to evaluate and manage such situations.

Eclampsia

Eclampsia is one of the most serious complications of pregnancy. It refers to the occurrence of seizures and/or coma in a person with preeclampsia. Preeclampsia is a multiorgan disorder characterized by high blood pressure (above 140/90 mmHg), proteinuria (>4 g/day), edema, hemo-concentration, liver dysfunction, and hyperuricemia. Preeclampsia tends to occur in about 2–8% of pregnancies. Preeclampsia and eclampsia tend to occur more frequently in underdeveloped countries. Obesity, chronic hypertension, and diabetes predispose to preeclampsia. Nulliparity and adolescent pregnancy are other important risk factors that are particularly relevant for women with epilepsy. About 5–8% of women with pre-eclampsia develop eclampsia. Eclampsia has a high mortality risk, ranging from 1.8 to 5%.

Severe throbbing headache is often the first symptom of eclampsia. Some patients may report a visual aura that precedes the headache. Nevertheless, a continuous and generalized intense headache with alteration of sensorium would indicate possible intracranial hemorrhage. Seizure is the distinctive feature of eclampsia. Typically eclamptic seizures tend to be generalized tonic–clonic convulsions, often preceded by focal twitching over the face. Seizures are generally brief but the postictal drowsiness may last longer. Persistent partial (focal) seizures may indicate structural lesions such as hemorrhage or infarct in an appropriate location. It can be difficult to distinguish eclamptic seizures from epileptic seizures, particularly if the woman also has a history of preexisting epilepsy. In the latter case, women experience their habitual seizures and these often have a focal onset or aura. The eclamptic seizures occur on a background of preeclampsia and the seizures are more often generalized tonic–clonic seizures or focal seizures with postictal deficits. These women often report severe headache prior to the seizures. Transient visual obscuration or blindness can occur as a result of the vasospasm. Persistent cortical blindness can occur due to infarct in the occipital lobe. Weakness of extremities or sensory deficits can also rarely occur. Postpartum eclampsia may not manifest the hypertension, pedal edema, or proteinuria that are characteristic of preeclampsia [2]. The causes of eclampsia in such instances are persistence of gestational hypertension, preeclampsia, or preexisting chronic hypertension [3].

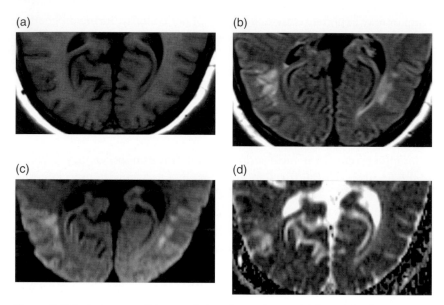

Figure 7.1 Posterior reversible encephalopathy syndrome. (a) T1-weighted image showing hypointensity in parieto-occipital region bilaterally. (b) FLAIR image showing hyperintensity in the corresponding area. (c) Diffusion-weighted image showing hyperintensity. (d) Corresponding apparent diffusion coefficient (ADC) image also showing hyperintensity, suggesting facilitated diffusion as seen in vasogenic edema.

Electroencephalography

Pregnancy per se does not lead to any changes in background activities on electroencephalography (EEG). The interictal findings in individuals with eclampsia include slowing of background activity (generalized or focal), intermittent spike and sharp-wave transients [4], and burst suppression pattern [5]. The EEG changes revert back to normal in a week's time in most cases.

Brain imaging

Brain imaging offers valuable data that can help in the diagnosis and prognostication. Reversible changes including hypodensity in the occipital lobes and subependymal bleed have been described with computed tomography (CT) of the brain soon after eclamptic seizures [6]. The characteristic changes on MRI in eclampsia include features of posterior reversible leukoencephalopathy (Figure 7.1). These changes may be due to alterations in regional cerebral hemodynamics and endothelial damage. Unlike other causes of posterior reversible leukoencephalopathy, those with eclampsia tend to have more headache and relatively normal mental status. There is less involvement of thalamus and basal ganglia and less cerebral edema in eclampsia [7]. Diffusion-weighted MRI can be useful in eclampsia as it can distinguish between vasogenic and cytotoxic

Table 7.2 WHO recommended interventions for prevention or treatment of preeclampsia and eclampsia.

Recommendation	Quality of evidence	Strength of recommendation
In areas where dietary calcium intake is low, calcium supplementation during pregnancy (1.5–2.0 g elemental calcium daily) is recommended for the prevention of preeclampsia in all women, but especially those at high risk of developing preeclampsia	Moderate	Strong
Women with severe hypertension during pregnancy should receive treatment with antihypertensive drugs	Very low	Strong
Magnesium sulfate is recommended for the prevention of eclampsia in women with severe preeclampsia in preference to other anticonvulsants	High	Strong
Magnesium sulfate is recommended for the treatment of women with eclampsia in preference to other anticonvulsants	Moderate	Strong
The full intravenous or intramuscular magnesium sulfate regimens are recommended for the prevention and treatment of eclampsia	Moderate	Strong
In women with severe preeclampsia at term, early delivery is recommended	Low	Strong

Source: adapted with permission from *WHO Recommendations for Prevention and Treatment of Pre-eclampsia and Eclampsia.* Geneva: World Health Organization, 2011.

edema [8]. The precise prevalence and diagnostic specificity of these findings have not been ascertained.

Treatment

There has been a long-standing debate about the ideal drugs to manage seizures in eclampsia. Magnesium sulfate had been widely used in the USA, while phenytoin or diazepam has been popular in Europe and several other countries. Recent international multicenter studies that compared the efficacy and adverse effects of these regimens have shown that magnesium sulfate is superior to other treatments. Based on extensive review of the literature and evidence base, the World Health Organization has recommended several guidelines for treatment of severe preeclampsia and eclampsia (Table 7.2). Early delivery may be necessary if preeclampsia occurs before fetal viability is achieved, or if it occurs near term.

Posterior reversible encephalopathy syndrome

Posterior reversible encephalopathy syndrome (PRES) has been reported in the context of hypertensive encephalopathy, eclampsia, lupus nephritis, glomerulonephritis, immunosuppressive therapy with organ transplantation, and therapy with cyclosporine, tacrolimus and inter- feron alpha. The typical MRI findings include large areas of hyperintense signals in the white matter of occipital and parietal lobes. These lesions are hypointense or isointense on diffusion-weighted images, with increased apparent diffusion coefficient suggestive of vasogenic edema. Mild involvement of the cerebral cortex may also be seen [9]. Although the imaging changes are characteristically located in the posterior head region, other locations can also be affected: frontal lobes (68%), inferior temporal lobes (40%), cerebellar hemispheres (30%), basal ganglia (14%), brainstem (13%), and deep white matter (18%) including the splenium (10%) [10]. A rare cause of PRES can be inadvertent dural puncture for cesarean section [11].

Reversible cerebral vasoconstriction syndrome

Reversible cerebral vasoconstriction syndrome is a rare disorder that can present as thunderclap headaches in the postpartum period. Patients can develop subarachnoid or parenchymal bleed manifesting as acute headache, alteration of sensorium, seizures, neck stiffness, or focal neurological signs. This often is misdiagnosed as cerebral venous sinus thrombosis or acute stroke in the postpartum period. Cerebral angiogram shows segmental reversible vasoconstriction (Figure 7.2). High-resolution contrast-enhanced MRI of the cerebral arteries may distinguish reversible vasospasm (no enhancement of the vessel wall) from vasculitis or cocaine angiopathy which may show enhancement [12]. Calcium channel blockers like verapamil can be used intravenously or intraarterially to manage reversible cerebral vasoconstriction syndrome.

Stroke during pregnancy

Acute arterial or venous strokes are important causes of seizures in pregnancy and the postpartum period [13]. The estimated prevalence of acute peripartum stroke is 13.1 and postpartum venous thrombosis 11.6 per 100 000 deliveries [14]. Seizure may be the only symptom of acute stroke when it affects relatively silent areas of the brain. In certain instances, it may be difficult to distinguish postictal weakness from acute

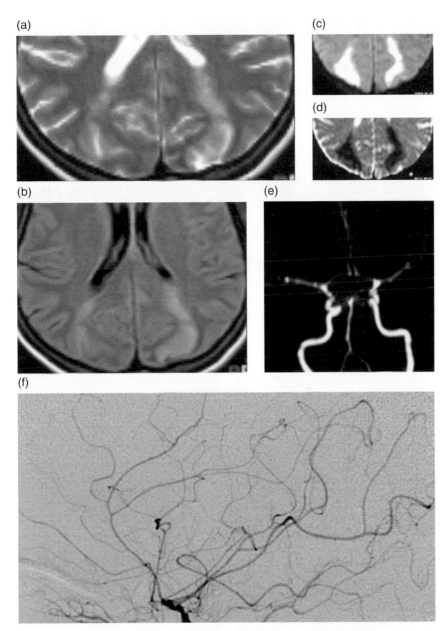

Figure 7.2 Reversible cerebral vasoconstriction syndrome. (a) Homogeneous hyperintensity in T2-weighted image, (b) FLAIR, (c) diffusion-weighted image showing hyperintensity in same location with (d) restricted ADC values. (e) Magnetic resonance angiogram showed multiple areas of irregular narrowing with a beaded appearance. (f) Digital subtraction angiography done 2 weeks later showed reversibility of beaded appearance, but the diffuse vasospasm was persisting.

stroke but diffusion and perfusion MRI can help to identify infarcted areas from vasogenic edema or ischemia. There are several pregnancy-specific causes for acute stroke (see Table 7.1).

Cerebral venous thrombosis

Typically, women with cerebral venous thrombosis (CVT) present with headache, seizures, alteration of sensorium, or focal deficits in the postpartum period, mostly beyond the third postpartum day but about 10% can present in the antepartum period. Patients with pregnancy-associated CVT may have prothrombotic markers such as dehydration, polymorphism of methylenetetrahydrofolate reductase and factor V genes, elevated levels of factor VIII, and abnormalities of other proteins associated with coagulation [15]. CVT has characteristic imaging findings [16]. Thrombosis of the superior sagittal sinus and/or its cortical draining veins are seen in two-thirds of women, while in the other third the deeper system of veins are affected alone or in combination with other sinuses. T1 and T2 MRI sequences, echoplanar susceptibility weighted T2 images, FLAIR and magnetic resonance venography confirm the diagnosis of CVT in most cases (Figure 7.3).

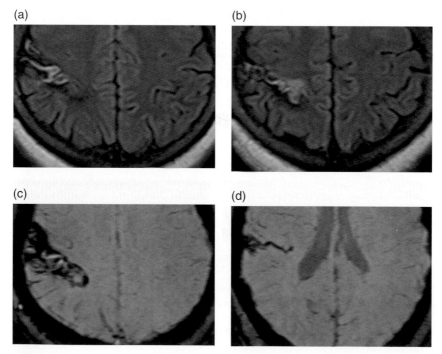

Figure 7.3 Cerebral venous sinus thrombosis showing linear FLAIR hyperintensity in the right precentral region (a, b) and susceptibility-weighted images showing peripheral blooming (c) and a cord-like hypointensity corresponding to the thrombosed cortical vein, i.e., cord sign (d).

The treatment of acute CVT includes anticoagulation with subcutaneous fractionated heparin or intravenous heparin. Raised intracranial pressure, seizures and headache due to CVT are managed according to established lines of management.

Vascular malformations
Arteriovenous malformation

Arteriovenous malformations (AVMs) are fistulous connections of arteries and veins without a normal intervening capillary bed [17]. Cerebral AVMs present with intracranial bleed (38–65%), seizures (15–35%), headache (15%), or neurological deficits (<10%). Nevertheless, they can also be asymptomatic in as many as 40% of people. Cerebral hemorrhage during pregnancy is the third leading cause of maternal death from nonobstetric causes. Eclampsia, rupture of AVM or aneurysm, venous thrombosis, hypertension, and choriocarcinoma are the leading causes of intracerebral bleed during pregnancy (Figure 7.4).

Cerebral AVM can be a matter of great concern during pregnancy. There is some controversy regarding the risk of rupture of AVM during pregnancy.

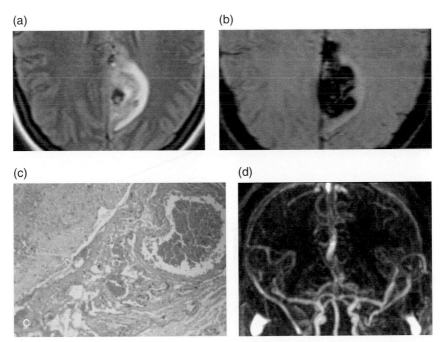

Figure 7.4 Arteriovenous malformation. (a) FLAIR image showing hyperintensity with central hypointensity. (b) Susceptibility-weighted image showing blooming suggestive of bleed. (c) Histopathology of the resected specimen (H&E stain, ×200) shows clusters of vascular channels of varying sizes, composed of dilated veins and thick-walled arterioles. (d) Magnetic resonance angiogram failed to demonstrate the arteriovenous malformation.

Robinson *et al.* [18] have shown that women with AVMs have a higher risk of a bleed during pregnancy or afterwards. It should be noted that these authors used a wider definition of pregnancy that included a period of 2 years after delivery. The risk of rebleeding during a subsequent pregnancy is high if a woman with an AVM had a bleed during the previous pregnancy. Horton *et al.* [19] studied 540 pregnancies in 451 women with AVMs, of which only 17 pregnancies were complicated by hemorrhage (3.15%; 95% CI 1.97–4.98). In this study, the risk of a bleed during pregnancy was comparable (3.5%) to that during the nongravid period for those with no history of a bleed. Those who had hemorrhage prior to pregnancy carried a higher risk (5.8%) of a bleed during pregnancy. These results cannot be generalized for all women with AVMs as the sample consisted of those with smaller lesions who were considered for proton beam therapy. The risk of a bleed from an AVM tends to increase in the latter half of pregnancy and labor (due to increased perfusion through the AVM as cerebral flow increases and due to increased straining, respectively). Nevertheless, normal delivery has been reported in many patients. AVM with acute bleed during pregnancy can be managed with endovascular intervention without jeopardizing fetal health in order to prevent further bleeding during pregnancy. The AVM can be excised after delivery in such instances [20].

Cavernous angioma

Cavernous angioma often presents as seizures in young women. Similar to AVM the risk of a bleed from a cavernous angioma may increase during pregnancy [21].

Postpartum cerebral angiopathy

Postpartum cerebral angiopathy [22] often mimics postpartum eclampsia. In a recent series of 18 patients with postpartum cerebral angiopathy, 28% presented with seizures. Other symptoms included headache, focal signs, visual disturbance, and encephalopathy. Their symptoms started around the end of the first week after delivery and about two-thirds had experienced an uneventful pregnancy. Half of them made a complete recovery while others had a fatal outcome (22%) or fixed deficits (28%). Cerebral vasospasm is demonstrated by angiography. Nimodipine or intraarterial nicardipine is used to treat this condition. There is an overlap between reversible cerebral vasoconstriction syndrome and postpartum cerebral angiopathy.

Amniotic fluid embolism

Amniotic fluid embolism is another rare complication, seen in 1 in 8000 to 1 in 80 000 pregnancies. It carries a high maternal and fetal mortality.

It presents as severe hypotension, acute respiratory distress syndrome, seizures, disseminated intravascular coagulation, and severe fetal distress during labor. About half have seizures as the presenting manifestation [23]. Initially it was considered that amniotic fluid embolism is a complication of prolonged and tumultuous labor, but it can occur in normal delivery or after cesarean section. Current research indicates that the syndrome is more of a maternal immunological response to the presence of amniotic fluid and fetal debris in the maternal circulation and lungs [24]. Patients are usually managed in critical care units with supportive measures and seizures are managed as for status epilepticus.

Central nervous system infections

Acute encephalitis or other central nervous system (CNS) infections are important causes of seizures during pregnancy. Fever, headache, alteration of sensorium, seizures, and focal deficits are the major clinical features of encephalitis. A variety of viral, bacterial, and protozoal encephalitides have been described during pregnancy. Immunological status, epidemiological factors, or exposure to vectors determine the precise cause of encephalitis. Brain abscess, tuberculoma, and listeriosis are other CNS infections that may present with seizures during pregnancy.

Neurocysticercosis

Neurocysticercosis is an infection in which the larval form of *Taenia solium* (pork tapeworm) gets lodged in the brain and leads to seizures, headache, and symptoms of raised intracranial pressure. Nevertheless, seizure is the presenting manifestation of neurocysticercosis in over two-thirds of cases. Humans are the definitive host for *Taenia*. Adult worms remain in the intestine and release eggs (proglottids) that pass out with the feces. In neurocysticercosis, humans are infected through fecal–oral contamination and the eggs transform to larvae which become deposited in the brain and other soft tissues. In endemic areas neurocysticercosis accounts for 25% or higher proportion of epilepsy cases and is a very common cause of seizures during pregnancy [25]. The diagnosis of neurocysticercosis is based on imaging findings (small cystic lesions with scolex or typical calcifications visible on MRI or CT of head), positive enzyme-linked immune electrotransfer blot (EITB), and epidemiological features (exposure to *T. solium* by travel or living in endemic areas). Albendazole 15 mg/kg daily for 1–3 weeks is generally recommended. Albendazole is a category C drug that can cause fetal malformations and is generally avoided during pregnancy. It may be used during pregnancy only if the benefits clearly outweigh the risk of malformation.

(a)

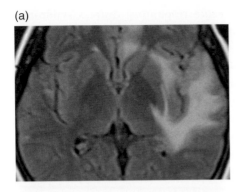

(b)

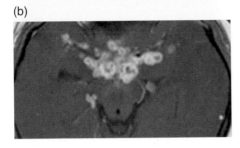

Figure 7.5 Tuberculoma. MRI FLAIR image showing extensive areas of hyperintensity in basifrontal and left temporal lobe (a) and multiple conglomerate ring-enhancing lesions of variable size in the suprasellar and perimesenchephalic cisterns (b).

Tuberculoma

Seizure is the presenting manifestation of CNS tuberculoma in more than half the cases. It can exacerbate during pregnancy (Figure 7.5) [26,27]. Multidrug-resistant variants of tuberculoma have become an emerging problem in the recent past.

Autoimmune encephalitis

Acute encephalitis-like presentation of seizures with altered sensorium during pregnancy can be due to autoimmune encephalitis. Autoimmune encephalitis is often mistaken for infective encephalitis and is under-recognized. However, this etiology should be considered and excluded particularly when the laboratory tests for infective etiologies are negative. The autoantibodies associated with encephalitis can be against intracytoplasmic antigens (limbic encephalitis [28], late-onset Rasmussen encephalitis [29]) or neuronal membrane antigens (*N*-methyl-D-aspartate receptor [30], voltage-gated potassium channels, and GluR3). Seizures can be a presenting manifestation for systemic autoimmune disorders such as systemic lupus erythematosus [31,32], antiphospholipid antibodies, anticardiolipin and anti-β_2-glycoprotein I antibodies [33], and Hashimoto encephalopathy. Unlike other forms of encephalitis, the seizures of autoimmune encephalitis respond better to steroids than to AEDs.

Brain tumors

Brain tumors are rather rare during pregnancy. Gliomas and meningiomas constitute 30% each of the brain tumors presenting during pregnancy. The role of reproductive ovarian hormones on the genesis of these tumors is uncertain, although they are known to express receptors to progesterone, estrogen, and androgen [34]. These tumors may present during pregnancy as seizures, raised intracranial pressure, or neurological deficits. The clinical status of the patient may acutely aggravate during pregnancy because of the tendency to retain water and electrolytes during pregnancy [35].

Diagnostic approach

History
A woman presenting with seizures during pregnancy is a medical emergency. A history of unprovoked seizures prior to pregnancy, use of AEDs or previous evaluation for seizures would suggest an epileptic syndrome. Past history of epilepsy needs to be confidentially elicited, as in several geographic areas women with epilepsy may not disclose their condition to the spouse or to the emergency physicians for fear of the stigma. Noncompliance with medications (for fear of fetal malformation or other reasons), sleep deprivation, mental stress, and hyperemesis gravidarum interfering with oral AED administration are some of the factors that predispose to relapse of seizures during early pregnancy in previously controlled epilepsy. Details of the precise AED usage are important as the blood levels of some of these drugs, particularly lamotrigine, oxcarbazepine and phenytoin, can drop considerably in the later stages of pregnancy. History of hypertension, proteinuria, or edema would point to the possibility of eclampsia as the cause of seizures. History of contact with tuberculosis, travel or stay in endemic areas of cysticercosis, fever, alteration of sensorium, or dehydration would help the physician to narrow down the differential diagnosis to CNS infections or CVT. A history of substance abuse and alcohol use during pregnancy is important for the diagnosis. The seizure semiology can also help to distinguish a habitual complex partial seizure of mesial temporal lobe epilepsy from eclamptic seizures, which often tend to be generalized tonic–clonic seizures preceded by multifocal twitching.

Examination
The physical examination should record the blood pressure, pedal edema, dermal vasculitic changes, or markers of infection (fever, lymphadenopathy)

or substance abuse. Persistent alteration of sensorium, papilledema, focal neurological signs, or meningeal signs are important in distinguishing various causes of seizures during pregnancy. Occasionally it can be difficult to distinguish eclampsia from CVT, cerebritis or encephalitides. Laboratory evidence of preeclampsia such as proteinuria and hyperuricemia can help in confirming eclampsia.

New-onset seizures generally require brain imaging. In the nonpregnant state this work-up may include CT, MRI, and occasionally digital subtraction angiography. These investigations are generally avoided during pregnancy. CT of the head can nevertheless be carried out if the benefits far outweigh the risk. With modern scanners, the radiation exposure to the fetus is less than 0.005 mGy, a radiation dose that is acceptable from a safety viewpoint. It is customary to cover the abdomen with lead apron when the mother undergoes cranial CT. MRI is not known to cause any fetal damage. The contrast agents used during the imaging can be another source of concern with regard to fetal safety. MRI of the brain can provide valuable information about the underlying cerebral pathology. Cerebral tumors, abscess, cerebritis, bleed, enhancing lesions, vascular malformations, tuberculoma, and cysticercus granuloma can be identified with a plain and contrast sequence of MRI. Diffusion-weighted images and apparent diffusion coefficient (ADC) maps can help to distinguish vasogenic edema from infarcts and cytotoxic edema as in the case of eclampsia and PRES.

EEG will be of use for exploring the electroclinical correlation in pregnant women with seizures. Juvenile myoclonic epilepsy can present for the first time during pregnancy, and characteristic generalized fast atypical spike–wave discharges, photoparoxysmal response, and normal background activity would support that diagnosis. Patients with eclampsia or PRES may have focal or generalized slowing of the background and rarely epileptiform discharges. EEG can also be of use while treating status epilepticus during pregnancy.

Review of the case: With regard to the case presented, the young age and new-onset seizures in the postpartum period on a background of preeclampsia initially favors a diagnosis of eclampsia. Nevertheless, the occurrence of seizures after the first two postpartum days, characteristic focal seizures with postictal deficits, and poor response to magnesium sulfate make that diagnosis unlikely. MRI and magnetic resonance venography confirmed CVT. Clinicians need to keep an open mind and search for the precise cause of seizures during pregnancy even when the woman has preexisting seizures. It is important to take urgent measures to control seizures, particularly generalized tonic–clonic seizures. Neurologists should work along with the gynecologist and neonatologists as a team while managing seizures during pregnancy and the peripartum period.

Key summary points

- Seizures can occur during pregnancy for several reasons, including new-onset epilepsy.

- Detailed history, physical examination, and appropriate imaging help the physician to reach a precise diagnosis in most situations.

- Seizures during pregnancy require emergency management for the safety of the mother and fetus.

References

1 Thomas SV, Syam U, Devi JS. Predictors of seizures during pregnancy in women with epilepsy. *Epilepsia* 2012;53:e85–e88.

2 Lubarsky SL, Barton JR, Friedman SA, Nasreddine S, Ramadan MK, Sibai BM. Late postpartum eclampsia revisited. *Obstet Gynecol* 1994;83:502–505.

3 Sibai BM. Etiology and management of postpartum hypertension–preeclampsia. *Am J Obstet Gynecol* 2012;206:470–475.

4 Thomas SV, Somanathan N, Radhakumari R. Interictal EEG changes in eclampsia. *Electroencephalogr Clin Neurophysiol* 1995;94:271–275.

5 Moodley J, Bobat SM, Hoffman M, Bill PL. Electroencephalogram and computerised cerebral tomography findings in eclampsia. *Br J Obstet Gynaecol* 1993;100:984–988.

6 Thomas SV, Somanathan N, Rao VR, Radhakurmari K. Reversible non enhancing lesions without focal neurological deficits in eclampsia. *Indian J Med Res* 1996;103: 94–97.

7 Liman TG, Bohner G, Heuschmann PU, Scheel M, Endres M, Siebert E. Clinical and radiological differences in posterior reversible encephalopathy syndrome between patients with preeclampsia–eclampsia and other predisposing diseases. *Eur J Neurol* 2012;19:935–943.

8 Schaefer PW, Buonanno FS, Gonzalez RG, Schwamm LH. Diffusion-weighted imaging discriminates between cytotoxic and vasogenic edema in a patient with eclampsia. *Stroke* 1997;28:1082–1085.

9 Lamy C, Oppenheim C, Méder JF, Mas JL. Neuroimaging in posterior reversible encephalopathy syndrome. *J Neuroimaging* 2004;14:89–96.

10 Bartynski WS, Boardman JF. Distinct imaging patterns and lesion distribution in posterior reversible encephalopathy syndrome. *AJNR Am J Neuroradiol* 2007;28:1320–1327.

11 Minai FN, Hasan SF, Sheerani M. Post-dural puncture posterior reversible encephalopathy syndrome. *J Coll Physicians Surg Pak* 2011;21:37–39.

12 Mandell DM, Matouk CC, Farb RI *et al.* Vessel wall MRI to differentiate between reversible cerebral vasoconstriction syndrome and central nervous system vasculitis: preliminary results. *Stroke* 2012;43:860–862.

13 Sidorov EV, Feng W, Caplan LR. Stroke in pregnant and postpartum women. *Expert Rev Cardiovasc Ther* 2011;9:1235–1247.

14 Lanska DJ, Kryscio RJ. Risk factors for peripartum and postpartum stroke and intracranial venous thrombosis. *Stroke* 2000;31:1274–1282.

15 Aaron S, Alexander M, Maya T *et al.* Underlying prothrombotic states in pregnancy associated cerebral venous thrombosis. *Neurol India* 2010;58:555–559.

16 Bousser MG, Ferro JM. Cerebral venous thrombosis: an update. *Lancet Neurol* 2007;6:162–170.

17 Fleming KD, Brown RD Jr. The natural history of intracranial vascular malformations. In: Winn HR (ed.) *Youman's Neurological Surgery*, 6th edn. Amsterdam: Elsevier, 2011: 4016–4033.

18 Robinson JL, Hall CS, Sedzimir CB. Arteriovenous malformations, aneurysms, and pregnancy. *J Neurosurg* 1974;41:63–70.

19 Horton JC, Chambers WA, Lyons SL, Adams RD, Kjellberg RN. Pregnancy and the risk of hemorrhage from cerebral arteriovenous malformations. *Neurosurgery* 1990;27:867–871.

20 Dashti SR, Spalding AC, Yao TL. Multimodality treatment of a ruptured grade IV posterior fossa arteriovenous malformation in a patient pregnant with twins: case report. *J Neurointerv Surg* 2012;4:e21.

21 Raychaudhuri R, Batjer HH, Awad IA. Intracranial cavernous angioma: a practical review of clinical and biological aspects. *Surg Neurol* 2005;63:319–328.

22 Fugate JE, Ameriso SF, Ortiz G *et al*. Variable presentations of postpartum angiopathy. *Stroke* 2012;43:670–676.

23 Gist RS, Stafford IP, Leibowitz AB, Beilin Y. Amniotic fluid embolism. *Anesth Analg* 2009;108:1599–1602.

24 Benson MD. Current concepts of immunology and diagnosis in amniotic fluid embolism. *Clin Dev Immunol* 2012;(2012): Article no. 946576.

25 Pandian JD, Venkateswaralu K, Thomas SV, Sarma PS. Maternal and fetal outcome in women with epilepsy associated with neurocysticercosis. *Epileptic Disord* 2007;9:285–291.

26 Ahmadi SA, Roozbeh H, Abbasi A, Bahadori M, Moghaddam KG, Ketabchi SE.Cerebral tuberculoma in pregnancy: overview of the literature and report of a case. *Acta Med Iran* 2011;49:64–69.

27 Liu C, Christie LJ, Neely J *et al*. Tuberculous meningoencephalitis in a pregnant woman presenting 7 years after removal of a cerebral granuloma. *Eur J Clin Microbiol Infect Dis* 2008;27:233–236.

28 Nishiyama K, Komori M, Narushima M, Yoshizawa H, Kawamata M, Ozaki M. A woman who required long-term mechanical ventilation to treat limbic encephalitis during pregnancy. *Acta Anaesthesiol Scand* 2007;51:252–254.

29 Larner AJ, Smith SJ, Duncan JS, Howard RS. Late-onset Rasmussen's syndrome with first seizure during pregnancy. *Eur Neurol* 1995;35:172.

30 Dalmau J, Lancaster E, Martinez-Hernandez E, Rosenfeld MR, Balice-Gordon R. Clinical experience and laboratory investigations in patients with anti-NMDAR encephalitis. *Lancet Neurol* 2011;10:63–74.

31 Borahay MA, Kelly BC, Harirah HM. Systemic lupus erythematosus presenting with leukocytoclastic vasculitis and seizure during pregnancy. *Am J Perinatol* 2009;26: 431–435.

32 El-Sayed YY, Lu EJ, Genovese MC, Lambert RE, Chitkara U, Druzin ML. Central nervous system lupus and pregnancy: 11-year experience at a single center. *J Matern Fetal Neonatal Med* 2002;12:99–103.

33 Shrivastava A, Dwivedi S, Aggarwal A, Misra R. Anti-cardiolipin and anti-beta2 glycoprotein I antibodies in Indian patients with systemic lupus erythematosus: association with the presence of seizures. *Lupus* 2001;10:45–50.

34 Wigertz A, Lönn S, Hall P *et al*. Reproductive factors and risk of meningioma and glioma. *Cancer Epidemiol Biomarkers Prev* 2008;17:2663–2670.

35 Olivi A, Bydon M, Raza SM. Brain tumours during pregnancy. In: Winn HR (ed.) *Youman's Neurological Surgery*, 6th edn. Amsterdam: Elsevier, 2011: 1229–1235.

CHAPTER 8

Seizure Control During Pregnancy

Anne Sabers

Epilepsy Clinic, Department of Neurology, University State Hospital – Rigshospitalet,
Copenhagen, Denmark

> **Case history:** *B.H. is a 35-year-old woman with generalized epilepsy who has been seizure-free for several years on lamotrigine 400 mg/day (200 mg + 200 mg) monotherapy. She was previously informed about the potential risk of seizure deterioration during pregnancy and due to her job situation, being dependent on the ability to drive a car, she was not willing to risk losing seizure control. For the same reason she would not consider discontinuation of antiepileptic medication.*

Background and details

Fortunately, most women with epilepsy can expect their seizure control to be unaffected by pregnancy. Women with epilepsy who want to have children probably represent the more healthy proportion of the female population with epilepsy, and the majority of these women have well-controlled epilepsy and are not restricted in their daily activities. For many of these women, seizure deterioration may pose serious consequences for their psychosocial life. Even a single breakthrough seizure may have implications for driving privileges and negatively influence the patient's self-esteem and family dynamics [1,2]. Poorly controlled tonic–clonic seizures can also cause miscarriage and affect maternal and fetal health [3].

The goal for the treatment of epilepsy during pregnancy is to obtain the best possible control of seizures with the least adverse effects for the mother and child. Therefore, the challenge for the physician and the therapeutic dilemma is to balance the risk of harmful effects associated with antiepileptic drug (AED) exposure to the developing fetus against the risk of therapeutic failure secondary to inadequate AED treatment. To determine

---

Epilepsy in Women, First Edition. Edited by Cynthia L. Harden, Sanjeev V. Thomas
and Torbjörn Tomson.

the best practical treatment strategy and ensure optimal seizure control throughout pregnancy, understanding the variability of gestational-induced pharmacokinetic alterations for individual AEDs is essential and is discussed in detail in Chapter 9.

Seizure control in pregnancy

Seizure activity during pregnancy has always been a matter of concern and is widely studied. The first reports were published in the nineteenth century, but results have varied considerably among the studies mainly due to methodological inconsistencies. The American Academy of Neurology (AAN) recently concluded that insufficient evidence currently exists to determine if changes in seizure frequency occur in pregnancy since an appropriate comparator group with nonpregnant women with epilepsy has never been included [4]. For the same reason, it is uncertain if status epilepticus occurs more frequently during pregnancy than during other periods of life. However, based on a number of observational studies, an increased seizure risk is found in approximately one-third to one-quarter of pregnant women with epilepsy. Results vary among the studies, particularly concerning which types of seizures are counted and how seizure changes during pregnancy are defined. Most studies have investigated seizure frequency changes during pregnancy in terms of worsened, unchanged, or improved seizure control compared with the 6–12 months prior to pregnancy. Only a few studies have reported absolute numbers of seizures and what these numbers might imply. "Increased seizure frequency" typically covers cases with an increased total number of seizures, but whether cases with a single seizure relapse are included is unclear. "Unchanged seizure frequency" typically reflects patients who have an unchanged number of seizures, which also includes patients who were seizure-free prior to pregnancy and continued to be seizure-free throughout pregnancy. "Reduced seizure frequency" generally covers patients who have a decreased number of seizures, but whether these cases include the mothers who regained complete seizure control after an unsuccessful attempt to withdraw AED treatment prior to pregnancy is unclear [5], or for women with very mild epilepsy and rare seizures, whether AEDs were discontinued temporarily in the first trimester to avoid teratogenic effects of AEDs during organogenesis.

The risk of a gestational-related increase in the number of seizures has been intensively discussed. In 1983, Schmidt [6] reviewed 27 studies published between 1884 and 1980 that included 2165 pregnancies and found that the average risk of increased seizure frequency was 24% (range 4–75%). A subsequent review of studies published from 1980 to 2006 and covering more than 4000 pregnancies found increased seizure frequency in 25% of cases (range 13–47%) [7]. Thus, it seems that the average risk of increased seizure frequency has remained relatively stable over more than 100 years despite the development of a wide array of AEDs and the substantial knowledge and awareness about AED pharmacokinetics that has emerged.

In most women pregnancy has no effect on their seizure frequency [5,8,9]. The largest prospective study of seizure control in pregnancy to date (the EURAP study) comprised 1736 women and reported that close to 60% of women with epilepsy remain seizure-free during pregnancy and, using the first trimester as a reference, seizure control was unchanged in 64% of the women [9].

Status epilepticus occurs in 1–2% of pregnancies in women with epilepsy and does not seem to be more frequent than in other periods of life. The EURAP study reported 36 cases of status epilepticus with one fetal death but no maternal fatalities [9].

Alterations in seizure control in different stages of pregnancy, labor, and delivery

The literature indicates some controversy about the worsening and improvement of seizures during different stages of gestation. Though most studies have shown that seizure deterioration occurs at the end of the pregnancy, other studies have found that a substantial number of cases experience an increase in the first trimester. The differences probably reflect random variation or spontaneous fluctuation in seizure occurrence in most cases, but specific psychological, pathophysiological, and pharmacokinetic aspects of certain drug regimens may also contribute [5, 9] (Table 8.1). Using the first trimester as a reference, no differences were found in the EURAP study between the second and third trimesters with respect to risk of deteriorated seizure control. Breakthrough seizures in

Table 8.1 Factors influencing seizure control during pregnancy.

Pharmacokinetic factors/decreased AED plasma concentration caused by
Decreased drug absorption
Increased volume of distribution
Increased hepatic metabolism
Increased renal clearance
Psychological factors
Noncompliance with medications
Increased stress and anxiety
Physiological factors
Sleep deprivation
Hormonal changes: increased estrogen/progesterone ratio

women who were seizure-free up until the pregnancy tend to occur most frequently during the first trimester for patients who may be noncompliant as a result of inadequate information [5].

Labor and delivery is apparently the period with the highest risk of seizures. The risk of having a generalized tonic–clonic seizure during labor is approximately 1–2% and, when taking all types of seizures together, 5% of women with epilepsy on average will experience a seizure during labor or within the first 24 hours after delivery [10–12]. This is up to nine times greater than the risk during pregnancy in general [13]. The only factor that is significantly associated with seizures during delivery is the occurrence of seizures earlier in pregnancy [9]. One study reported a significant increase in focal seizures during early puerperium [13].

Risk factors for deteriorated seizure control

Numerous physiological changes might influence seizure activity in pregnancy [5,14,15]. Patients who are seizure-free before pregnancy are less likely to experience seizure deterioration during pregnancy [16], whereas focal epilepsy and the use of polytherapy and some specific AEDs are associated with a higher risk of seizures during pregnancy [5,9]. An association between altered seizure frequency and a longer history of the maternal epilepsy may also exist [17]. However, each pregnancy tends to have its own seizure pattern, which cannot be predicted from the experiences of previous pregnancies. Therefore, even if a serious worsening of seizures occurs during one pregnancy, the woman does not need to be discouraged if she wants to become pregnant again.

Pregnancy can alter the pharmacokinetics of most AEDs. Drug bioavailability, distribution, and elimination may be altered at many levels and lead to a fall in the plasma concentration of the AED. This decrease in plasma concentration is the most common explanation for therapeutic failure in many pregnant women.

The EURAP study demonstrated that seizure activity in pregnancy to some extent depends on which AED is used [9]. This dependence has been most systematically evaluated for lamotrigine, which has evolved as a drug of first choice for pregnant women due to the low teratogenic potential. Lamotrigine metabolism is enhanced in pregnancy by induced activity of the UDP-glucuronosyltransferase (UGT)1A4 isoenzyme, which is responsible for more than 90% of hepatic glucuronidation of lamotrigine. This enhanced activity is probably induced by elevated concentrations of sex steroid hormones, which most likely increase the expression of UGT. Declining plasma concentrations are most likely correlated with increased seizure frequency. Several independent studies have shown that lamotrigine monotherapy is associated with increased seizure frequency during pregnancy for more than 40% of patients [9,18–20], which represents a twofold higher risk of worsening seizures compared to treatment with most other AEDs [21]. A prospective study of 53 pregnant women treated with lamotrigine demonstrated a clear correlation between declining plasma concentrations of lamotrigine and increased seizure frequency. A decrease in lamotrigine plasma concentration to 65% of the pre-pregnancy individualized pre-pregnancy target lamotrigine concentration is a significant predictor of seizure deterioration [18]. On average, lamotrigine clearance during pregnancy is two to three times higher than before pregnancy, and the clearance rate increases progressively until the 32nd week of gestation [20,22]. After delivery, the rate of lamotrigine elimination decreases rapidly, within days, reaching pre-pregnancy levels within the first 1–3 weeks after birth. The extent to which pregnancy affects lamotrigine elimination varies considerably among patients, which to some extent can be explained by polymorphisms in the gene that encodes UGT activity. Ethnicity, for example, appears to significantly affect enzyme activity [18]. In addition, specific exogenous factors can contribute; for example, comedication with valproate almost entirely eliminates the pregnancy-related increase in lamotrigine metabolism [23]. Based on the Australian Pregnancy Register, seizure control is significantly worse in women treated with lamotrigine compared with valproate or carbamazepine. Two cases of fetal loss were reported in conjunction with status epilepticus/prolonged seizures following valproate withdrawal and replacement with lamotrigine [24].

Oxcarbazepine is another glucuronidated AED that is significantly affected by pregnancy [5,9]. The EURAP study demonstrated that seizure activity during pregnancy is associated with treatment with oxcarbazepine, and the need for dosage adjustments is specifically associated with treatment with lamotrigine and oxcarbazepine [5,9]; using these two AEDs in combination may pose a specific risk for seizure deterioration [25]. The plasma concentration of the active form of oxcarbazepine (the monohydroxy derivative, MHD) declines by 36–50% in late pregnancy [26], which is less than the decrease observed for lamotrigine but substantial and associated with increased seizure frequency in more than 50% of the women [27].

The elimination of levetiracetam also seems to be significantly affected by pregnancy [28,29]. As levetiracetam is only marginally metabolized, the mechanism behind this effect remains to be clarified, but it is likely explained by an increased renal glomerular filtration rate in later stages of pregnancy [29]. However, the clinical relevance of this pharmacokinetic effect has not been clarified.

Therapeutic failures may also be a consequence of excessive nausea, hyperemesis gravidarum, and noncompliance. Intentional noncompliance has been well documented in the literature [30]. Because most women have concerns about the potentially harmful effects of medications taken during pregnancy, they often have an intuitive resistance to accept increases in the dosages of AEDs. One study demonstrated that patients who were followed in a specialized epilepsy clinic prior to conception and throughout pregnancy had a significantly lower risk of seizure deterioration during pregnancy (9%) than those who were referred and received specialized assistance after conception (32%) [5], which probably reflects the effect of better drug compliance and a lower risk of abrupt discontinuation of AEDs due to improved patient knowledge.

Sleep deprivation, anxiety, and stress provoked by the pregnancy may also influence seizure vulnerability [15]. Changes in sex hormones may also contribute; the ratio of estrogen (general proconvulsant effects) to progesterone (probably having both proconvulsant and anticonvulsant properties) increases during pregnancy, reaching its peak between weeks 8 and 16 [13].

Measures to reduce the risk of seizures during pregnancy

Although the association between pharmacokinetic alterations and changes in seizure control have not been explored systematically for all AEDs, it is reasonable to assume that declining active drug concentrations in pregnancy are associated with an increased risk of seizures. This reasoning is the justification for regular drug level monitoring during pregnancy for all AEDs for which alterations can be expected and for which plasma concentrations can be determined. However, some controversy has existed as to whether AED dose adjustment is required based on decreased plasma concentrations alone, particularly in the vulnerable pregnancy period when teratogenic potential exists in relation to higher doses of the drugs. Many have recommended that patients should be treated on the basis of clinical findings, i.e., changes in seizure control, not just changes in plasma concentrations. However, up to 80% of women who conceive [5] have been seizure-free for long periods of time leading up to pregnancy and, for many of these women, loss of seizure control may pose serious consequences for their everyday social life and it is not acceptable to wait for breakthrough seizures to increase the dose. Notably, the magnitude of plasma concentration alterations is very difficult to predict and all these issues, with pros and cons, have to be carefully discussed with patients for their individual decisions.

Therefore, a reasonable approach for women with well-controlled seizures, with some exceptions, is to check AED levels at baseline (before conception) and monthly, with dose adjustments to maintain an effective and stable level throughout pregnancy. This approach has been supported by the AAN practice guidelines, at least for women who are treated with lamotrigine, oxcarbazepine, levetiracetam, or phenytoin [4].

Implications for management

An algorithm for dose adjustment before, during, and after pregnancy has been suggested for treatment with lamotrigine [31], but it is probably applicable to all those AEDs for which plasma concentrations can be expected to alter during pregnancy. Ideally, the AED dose should be adjusted individually before pregnancy to the lowest effective dose, and the optimal plasma level should be determined and used as a reference concentration for the pregnancy. If the plasma concentration falls below this reference, the AED dose should be increased by 20–25% and the plasma concentration checked after 4–5 weeks. The procedure should be repeated every 4–5 weeks throughout pregnancy. If the plasma concentration is higher or has not fallen to below the reference, the dose should not be changed, but the plasma level should be redetermined after 4–5 weeks. This close monitoring of plasma concentration and adjusting the dosage to maintain stable plasma levels throughout pregnancy can reduce the risk of seizure deterioration to approximately 9%, at least for lamotrigine monotherapy [5].

In settings where therapeutic drug monitoring is unavailable, increasing the dose of some AEDs might be advisable, i.e., increasing the dose of lamotrigine and oxcarbazepine, and probably levetiracetam, by approximately 20–25% in both second and third trimester. For patients who are treated with phenytoin and valproate, which are both more than 90% protein-bound, the free levels of these drugs should be followed during pregnancy rather than the total levels.

The role of pre-conception counseling and patient education

Pre-conception counseling should be offered to all women who are considering pregnancy. A multidisciplinary approach is recommended involving the primary care physician, an obstetrician, an epileptologist/neurologist, and a specialized nurse. Among a number of important issues related to the pregnancy, the main aim of pre-conception counseling is to ensure that the woman is fully aware of any risks and benefits related to the AED treatment. The information is not always remembered by the patient, which highlights the need for regular repetition of this type of information [32]. The psychological effects of adequate patient education and counseling initiated prior to pregnancy may significantly influence the results. Many women intuitively worry about the potential adverse effects of the drug on the developing fetus and therefore might be noncompliant or reluctant to accept frequent dose increases if they are uncertain and insecure regarding the background for this advice. Some of these problems may be corrected and insecurity and misunderstandings prevented by systematic pre-pregnancy patient education and continued close contact between the patient and the caregivers throughout the pregnancy. Inclusion of specially trained epilepsy nurses for routine education during visits may also be useful. To lower the costs, and for a pragmatic approach, the woman can be seen by an epileptologist on the first visit after conception and every second visit thereafter she can be seen by an epilepsy nurse. For well-educated patients and patients who have been through this process before, some of the check-ups can be performed over the telephone. Some of the blood tests can be performed locally by the patient's general practitioner, and patients themselves can ensure that the blood test results reach the epilepsy clinic. In addition, telephone contact with the patient and handling, ordering, and sampling of blood tests can be done by epilepsy nurses. If the patient is informed at this point, the question of compliance is more easily resolved.

Review of the case: For our case B.H., the pre-pregnancy plasma level of lamotrigine was determined as a reference (28 μmol/L). When the pregnancy was recognized in week 7, she was seen in the epilepsy clinic and plasma level of lamotrigine was monitored in week 9, 14, 21, 28, 32, and 36. Following a decline in the plasma concentration below her pre-pregnancy reference level, the dose of lamotrigine was increased gradually to 300 mg + 200 mg; 300 mg + 300 mg; 400 mg + 400 mg; 500 mg + 500 mg; and 600 mg + 500 mg during the course of the pregnancy. The dose was reduced to 400 mg + 500 mg the day after delivery and gradually reduced to 300 mg + 200 mg within the first 2 weeks after birth. She remained seizure-free without side effects throughout pregnancy.

 Key summary points

1. The majority of women remain seizure-free throughout pregnancy.
2. Approximately 25% experience seizure deterioration during pregnancy.
3. Status epilepticus is not more frequent during pregnancy than in other periods of life.
4. Plasma levels of AEDs should be obtained before pregnancy as a reference for dosing adjustments during pregnancy.
5. Levels of AEDs should be obtained monthly throughout pregnancy.
6. A close and systematic monitoring paradigm throughout pregnancy may diminish the risk of seizure aggravation.
7. Adequate pre-pregnancy counseling is essential to increase the likelihood of maintained seizure control.

References

1 Canuet L, Ishii R, Iwase M *et al*. Factors associated with impaired quality of life in younger and older adults with epilepsy. *Epilepsy Res* 2009;83:58–65.

2 Hixson JD, Kirsch HE. The effects of epilepsy and its treatments on affect and emotion. *Neurocase* 2009;15:206–216.

3 Chen YH, Chiou HY, Lin HC, Lin HL. Affect of seizures during gestation on pregnancy outcomes in women with epilepsy. *Arch Neurol* 2009;66:979–984.

4 Harden CL, Hopp J, Ting TY *et al*. Management issues for women with epilepsy. Focus on pregnancy (an evidence-based review): I. Obstetrical complications and change in seizure frequency: Report of the Quality Standards Subcommittee and Therapeutics and Technology Assessment Subcommittee of the American Academy of Neurology and the American Epilepsy Society. *Epilepsia* 2009;50:1229–1236.

5 Sabers A. Influences on seizure activity in pregnant women with epilepsy. *Epilepsy Behav* 2009;15:230–234.

6 Schmidt D. The effect of pregnancy on the natural history of epilepsy. In: Janz D, Dam M, Bossi L, Helge H, Richens A, Schmidt D (eds) *Epilepsy, Pregnancy, and the Child*. New York: Raven Press, 1982: 3–14.

7 Battino D, Tomson T. Seizure control in pregnancy. In: Panayiotopoulos CP, Crawford P, Tomson T (eds) *Epilepsies in Girls and Women*. Oxford: Medicinae, 2008: 138–142.

8 Nakken KO, Lillestolen KM, Tauboll E, Engelsen B, Brodtkorb E. [Epilepsy and pregnancy: drug use, seizure control, and complications.] *Tidsskr Nor Laegeforen* 2006;126:2507–2510.

9 EURAP Study Group. Seizure control and treatment in pregnancy: observations from the EURAP epilepsy pregnancy registry. *Neurology* 2006;66:354–360.

10 Gjerde IO, Strandjord RE, Ulstein M. The course of epilepsy during pregnancy: a study of 78 cases. *Acta Neurol Scand* 1988;78:198–205.

11 Tomson T, Hiilesmaa V. Epilepsy in pregnancy. *Br Med J* 2007;335:769–773.

12 Thomas SV, Sindhu K, Ajaykumar B, Sulekha Devi PB, Sujamol J. Maternal and obstetric outcome of women with epilepsy. *Seizure* 2009;18:163–166.

13 Bardy AH, Teramo K, Hiilesmaa VK. Apparent clearance of phenytoin, phenobarbitone, primidone, and carbamazepine during pregnancy: results of the prospective Helsinki study. In: Janz D, Dam M, Bossi L, Helge H, Richens A, Schmidt D (eds) *Epilepsy, Pregnancy, and the Child* New York: Raven Press, 1982: 141–145.

14 Pennell PB. Antiepileptic drug pharmacokinetics during pregnancy and lactation. *Neurology* 2003;61(6 Suppl 2):S35–S42.

15 Brodtkorb E, Reimers A. Seizure control and pharmacokinetics of antiepileptic drugs in pregnant women with epilepsy. *Seizure* 2008;17:160–165.

16 Sabers A, Rogvi-Hansen B, Dam M *et al*. Pregnancy and epilepsy: a retrospective study of 151 pregnancies. *Acta Neurol Scand* 1998;97:164–170.

17 Vajda FJ, Hitchcock A, Graham J, O'Brien T, Lander C, Eadie M. Seizure control in antiepileptic drug-treated pregnancy. *Epilepsia* 2008;49:172–176.

18 Pennell PB, Peng L, Newport DJ *et al*. Lamotrigine in pregnancy: clearance, therapeutic drug monitoring, and seizure frequency. *Neurology* 2008;70:2130–2136.

19 Petrenaite V, Sabers A, Hansen-Schwartz J. Individual changes in lamotrigine plasma concentrations during pregnancy. *Epilepsy Res* 2005;65:185–188.

20 de Haan GJ, Edelbroek P, Segers J *et al*. Gestation-induced changes in lamotrigine pharmacokinetics: a monotherapy study. *Neurology* 2004;63:571–573.

21 Sabers A, Tomson T. Managing antiepileptic drugs during pregnancy and lactation. *Curr Opin Neurol* 2009;22:157–161.

22 Ohman I, Beck O, Vitols S, Tomson T. Plasma concentrations of lamotrigine and its 2-*N*-glucuronide metabolite during pregnancy in women with epilepsy. *Epilepsia* 2008;49:1075–1080.

23 Tomson T, Luef G, Sabers A, Pittschieler S, Ohman I. Valproate effects on kinetics of lamotrigine in pregnancy and treatment with oral contraceptives. *Neurology* 2006;67:1297–1299.

24 Vajda FJ, Hitchcock A, Graham J *et al*. Foetal malformations and seizure control: 52 months data of the Australian Pregnancy Registry. *Eur J Neurol* 2006;13:645–654.

25 Wegner I, Edelbroek P, de Haan GJ, Lindhout D, Sander JW. Drug monitoring of lamotrigine and oxcarbazepine combination during pregnancy. *Epilepsia* 2010;51:2500–2502.

26 Christensen J, Sabers A, Sidenius P. Oxcarbazepine concentrations during pregnancy: a retrospective study in patients with epilepsy. *Neurology* 2006;67:1497–1499.

27 Petrenaite V, Sabers A, Hansen-Schwartz J. Seizure deterioration in women treated with oxcarbazepine during pregnancy. *Epilepsy Res* 2009;84:245–249.

28 Tomson T, Palm R, Kallen K *et al*. Pharmacokinetics of levetiracetam during pregnancy, delivery, in the neonatal period, and lactation. *Epilepsia* 2007;48:1111–1116.

29 Westin AA, Reimers A, Helde G, Nakken KO, Brodtkorb E. Serum concentration/dose ratio of levetiracetam before, during and after pregnancy. *Seizure* 2008;17:192–198.

30 Schmidt D, Canger R, Avanzini G *et al*. Change of seizure frequency in pregnant epileptic women. *J Neurol Neurosurg Psychiatry* 1983;46:751–755.

31 Sabers A. Algorithm for lamotrigine dose adjustment before, during, and after pregnancy. *Acta Neurol Scand* 2012;126:e1–e4.

32 Bell GS, Nashef L, Kendall S *et al*. Information recalled by women taking antiepileptic drugs for epilepsy: a questionnaire study. *Epilepsy Res* 2002;52:139–146.

CHAPTER 9

Effect of Pregnancy on AED Kinetics

Peter B. Forgacs[1] and Page B. Pennell[2]

[1]Rockefeller University, New York, New York, USA

[2]Division of Epilepsy, Harvard Medical School, Brigham and Women's Hospital, Boston, Massachusetts, USA

Case history: *K.L.M. was a 32 year-old right-handed G3P2 woman who presented to clinic at 10.5 weeks gestational age (GA) with a history of focal epilepsy since age 17 years. She described auras of "dream-like" feeling, followed by staring, oral automatisms, and postictal sleepiness. She had one generalized tonic–clonic seizure prior to medications. Her seizures were controlled on another antiepileptic drug (AED), but she was transitioned to lamotrigine in preparation for pregnancy at age 27 years old. Pre-conception dose was 650 mg/day with levels of 11–12 µg/mL, and she remained seizure-free. Her first pregnancy was complicated by lamotrigine toxicity. This was maximal post dose, manifested by dizziness and blurry vision, and occurred at 29 weeks GA while taking lamotrigine 1750 mg/day. No postpartum taper was prescribed and her ataxia recurred after delivery. Lamotrigine levels during this pregnancy and after birth were not available.*

Her second pregnancy was uneventful with no seizures or symptoms of lamotrigine toxicity; lamotrigine pre-conception dose was 650 mg/day with levels of 7.5–11.2 µg/mL. Maximal dose was 725 mg/day and empiric postpartum taper was prescribed. She presented to our clinic at 10.5 weeks GA with her third pregnancy on lamotrigine 650 mg/day. Lamotrigine level was 8.3 µg/mL. As new data suggested that level of fetal exposure may be important for all AEDs, it was decided to lower her individualized lamotrigine target concentration to 5–10 µg/mL and let her levels drift downward. She remained seizure-free. Maximal lamotrigine dose during late pregnancy was 800 mg/day. Her lamotrigine was tapered after birth to 650 mg/day, and she had no toxicity.

Introduction

In approximately 3–5 per 1000 childbirths, the child is born to a women with epilepsy [1]. Despite all the efforts of patient and physician education, a substantial number of women with epilepsy still have limited knowledge

---

Epilepsy in Women, First Edition. Edited by Cynthia L. Harden, Sanjeev V. Thomas and Torbjörn Tomson.

© 2013 John Wiley & Sons, Ltd. Published 2013 by John Wiley & Sons, Ltd.

of the possible teratogenic effects of AEDs [2]. The optimal management of epilepsy during pregnancy involves minimizing possible teratogenic side effects of AEDs while maintaining seizure freedom. Structural teratogenic risks have been described for virtually all the older and many of the newer AEDs [3–5]. Prenatal exposure to some AEDs can also affect cognition and behavior later in childhood [6,7]. It is also generally accepted that generalized tonic–clonic seizures and likely other seizure types are detrimental for the fetus and the mother [3,8]. There are multiple physiologic changes during pregnancy, which influence the pharmacokinetics of AEDs and therefore the plasma levels of certain medications. Knowledge and understanding of the magnitude and time course of these alterations is essential for the appropriate management of AEDs before, during, and after a pregnancy.

Implications of AED pharmacokinetics before pregnancy

Optimizing AED management before conception might improve seizure frequency during pregnancy [9,10]. The ideal goal for all women with epilepsy who are planning to become pregnant is to be on monotherapy [11] of an AED with the least teratogenic potential using the lowest effective dose [12,13]. The same ideal goal is desirable for all women who are at childbearing age, as teratogenic side effects of some AEDs might affect the fetus during the first few weeks of gestation, even before the pregnancy is discovered. In addition, about 50% of pregnancies in the USA are unplanned [14]. Medication dose adjustments and measurement of AED plasma levels in order to determine the individual's optimal target concentration should be achieved prior to pregnancy [9].

Oral contraceptives might affect the pharmacokinetics of certain AEDs and should be considered during pregnancy planning [15,16]. Estradiol-containing contraceptives increase the metabolism of AEDs that undergo glucuronidation, e.g., lamotrigine [17], valproate [18], and likely oxcarbazepine (Table 9.1). Some experts recommend measurement of AED plasma concentrations after hormonal contraceptives are discontinued, with subsequent dosage adjustments if possible to avoid unnecessary fetal exposure to higher, and potentially more teratogenic, AED levels [13,19,20].

It is important to determine the optimal effective medication concentration before the pregnancy. There is evidence that breakthrough seizures tend to occur when AED levels are subtherapeutic during pregnancy [21]. A prospective study found an association between seizure worsening and decrease in lamotrigine level to less than 65% compared

Table 9.1 Major routes of elimination of AEDs.

Renal excretion*
Levetiracetam
Pregabalin
Vigabatrin
Topiramate
Glucuronidation*
Valproate[†]
Lamotrigine
Oxcarbazepine
Cytochrome P450 metabolism[†]
Phenytoin[†]
Phenobarbital[†]
Carbamazepine[†]
Zonisamide

*Main route of metabolism.
[†]Highly protein bound.

with the patient's individual target concentration, ideally determined prior to conception [22]. There are limited studies about the significance of levels of other newer AEDs and seizure worsening during pregnancy, although the general consensus is that at least one but preferably two serum concentrations should be measured before the pregnancy when seizure control is optimal, for future comparison [12].

Pharmacokinetic changes during pregnancy

General aspects

There are a number of physiologic changes during pregnancy that affect the pharmacokinetics of AEDs. These include changes in absorption and bio-availability, modified drug distribution due to increased plasma volume and altered protein binding, increased renal excretion, and changes in liver metabolism through hepatic enzyme induction [23]. *Clearance* is a term used to encompass all these physiologic changes. A common simple formula is:

Clearance = daily dose(mg/kg)/AED concentration

In other words, clearance is a measure of how much AED daily dose is needed to maintain a certain concentration. Clearance increases for many of the AEDs during pregnancy, often beginning in the first trimester, with further increased clearance as the pregnancy progresses until delivery (Table 9.2).

Absorption of AEDs during pregnancy can be affected by changes in appetite and diet, the ability to maintain adequate nutrition, and alteration

Table 9.2 Alterations in AED clearance and/or total and free concentrations during pregnancy.

	Reported increases in total and free clearance	Reported decreases in total and free concentrations	Important remarks	Reference
Phenytoin	Total: 19–150% Free: 25% in TM3	Total: 25–70% Free: 16–31% in TM3		25, 30, 31
Carbamazepine	Total: −11 to +27%	Total: 0–12% Free: no change		25, 33, 34
Phenobarbital	Total: 60%	Total: 55% Free: 50%		31, 35, 36
Primidone	Inconsistent	Inconsistent	Decrease in derived phenobarbital concentrations, with lower phenobarbital/primidone ratios	39
Valproic acid	Total: Increased by TM2 and TM3 Free: no change	Free fraction increased by TM2 and TM3		37, 38
Ethosuximide	Inconsistent	Inconsistent		40
Lamotrigine	Total: 65–264%, substantial interindividual variability Free: 89%		Greater in whites compared with African-Americans Decrease in lamotrigine clearance by third week after birth	22, 41–45, 47
Oxcarbazepine	38.2%	MHD and active moiety decreased by 36–61%		48–51
Levetiracetam	243%	38–60% by TM3	Clearance back to baseline within the first few weeks after birth Significant interindividual variability noted	52–55
Topiramate	34–72%	40%	Pronounced interindividual variability noted	56, 57
Zonisamide	Increase in clearance peaks around 27 weeks' gestation	Over 50% decrease by 27 weeks' gestation		58
Tiagabine Pregabalin, vigabatrin		Considerable effect on plasma levels is expected Decrease is expected, but substantial interindividual variations are possible	No studies or case reports available No studies or case reports available	

MHD, monohydroxy derivative of oxcarbazepine; TM, trimester.

Source: adapted and modified from Pennell PB, Hovinga CA. Antiepileptic drug therapy in pregnancy I: gestation-induced effects on AED pharmacokinetics. *Int Rev Neurobiol* 2008;83:227–240.

in gastrointestinal bypass time. A significant problem for some patients is increased nausea and vomiting during pregnancy (i.e., hyperemesis gravidarum) with the inability to take or maintain oral medications in the gastrointestinal system for sufficient time for absorption. A case report [24] described a patient who developed status epilepticus secondary to decreased intestinal absorption of phenytoin.

AED distribution is affected by increased total body water and extracellular fluid volume and increased total body fat leading to decreased or at least altered elimination of lipid-soluble drugs. An important consideration for AEDs that are highly protein-bound (e.g., valproate, phenytoin, carbamazepine and phenobarbital) is the distribution between the free (unbound) and total (bound plus unbound) fraction of the medication (Table 9.1). During pregnancy, there is a decrease in the concentration of main plasma proteins, which results in decrease in total drug levels while the free and pharmacologically active fraction of these medications may be relatively less altered [19,25–27]. Therefore it is important to follow free plasma levels in addition to total levels for all AEDs that are highly protein-bound and when it is available [12].

Increased metabolism of certain AEDs is a major contributing factor to decreased AED concentration during pregnancy (Table 9.1). Major pathways of metabolism include induction of cytochrome P450 enzyme pathways (phenytoin, phenobarbital, carbamazepine), β-oxidation (valproate), and glucuronidation (valproate, lamotrigine, oxcarbazepine). Metabolism may increase up to two to three times compared with pre-pregnancy rates. These changes may rapidly reverse after delivery and may result in toxic levels of AEDs.

Excretion by the kidney is the major route of drug elimination for several AEDs (Table 9.1). Renal glomerular filtration rate and blood flow, in parallel with increased cardiac output, have an important potential role in decreased concentration of excreted AEDs. Levetiracetam levels are particularly decreased during the third trimester [28], although there are limited studies available for other renally excreted newer AEDs (pregabalin, vigabatrin, topiramate).

Pharmacokinetic changes detailed by medication
Phenytoin
Total phenytoin concentration decreases up to 25–70% during pregnancy, mostly secondary to increased hepatic metabolism through the cytochrome P450 system. Phenytoin is highly protein-bound, although free levels tend to decrease as well, albeit slightly less than total levels (16–31%) [25,29,30]. Total levels show the steepest decline during the first trimester, but are significantly lower during all three trimesters, while free levels tend to decrease less dramatically [31]. Lower phenytoin levels are associated with

increased seizure frequency, and therefore careful monitoring of total and free levels is recommended with appropriate increase in dose throughout the pregnancy [32].

Carbamazepine

Despite the pharmacokinetic properties of high protein binding and hepatic metabolism, studies revealed mixed results in carbamazepine level changes during pregnancy. One study showed a slight decrease during the second and third trimesters (9–12%) in the total levels, although free levels remained unchanged [25]. Other studies revealed minimal or no significant change in carbamazepine levels [33,34], but increase in carbamazepine epoxide levels and increased epoxide to carbamazepine ratios during pregnancy [35]. However, current guidelines recommend following carbamazepine levels during pregnancy due to the unpredictability of gestational-induced changes in total and free carbamazepine levels [32].

Phenobarbital, valproate, primidone and ethosuximide

Total and free phenobarbital levels are reported to decline up to 50–60% during pregnancy [35,36]. Total valproate levels also decrease significantly, although free levels change only minimally [37,38], while reports on primidone and ethosuximide levels are inconsistent [39,40]. Current recommendations render theses studies insufficient to provide enough information to determine predicted level changes of these AEDs during pregnancy; therefore, monitoring and following the level changes are encouraged.

Lamotrigine

Among the newer AEDs, pharmacokinetic changes are best characterized for lamotrigine in detail [22,41–43]. The vast majority (>90%) of lamotrigine is metabolized through glucuronidation, which is significantly enhanced during pregnancy likely secondary to increasing concentration of the sex steroid hormone estradiol [44]. However, in the first 2 months of pregnancy, the increase in renal excretion seems to be the major factor in increased clearance of lamotrigine [45]. Interaction with other AEDs that inhibit glucuronidation (e.g., valproate) needs to be considered as well, as lamotrigine level decrease could be minimal in these patients [46]. Lamotrigine clearance is reported to increase 65–264% during pregnancy, but significant individual variability is noted. A recent prospective observational study [22] reported total (94%) and free (89%) lamotrigine clearance is increased throughout pregnancy, peaking in the third trimester. Clearance was found to be significantly greater in white compared with black patients, suggesting that pharmacogenetics play a role in interindividual variability. Importantly, this study also reported that seizure frequency increased when lamotrigine levels decreased below 65% of the individualized target concentration, determined by pre-pregnancy levels. Another study demonstrated that close monitoring of lamotrigine levels with frequent dose adjustments decreased the risk of breakthrough seizures to 19% [47]. These studies provide strong evidence to support the current guidelines that lamotrigine levels should be frequently checked (at least monthly beginning at time of positive pregnancy test) and dosing should be appropriately changed during pregnancy [32].

Oxcarbazepine

Once ingested, oxcarbazepine quickly undergoes keto-reduction to an active monohydroxy derivative (MHD), which is subsequently metabolized by glucuronidation and to a lesser degree through renal excretion and cytochrome P450 metabolism. Two studies are available regarding the pharmacokinetic properties of oxcarbazepine, and these found that levels decreased by 36–61% by the third trimester [48,49]. One study found similar pharmacokinetic changes in oxcarbazepine and lamotrigine in patients who took both medications [50]. Another study showed that 8 of 14 patients on oxcarbazepine monotherapy had increased seizure frequency and found a trend toward correlation between worsening of seizures and decreased MHD concentrations [51]. More data are needed to sufficiently understand the pharmacokinetic changes of oxcarbazepine during pregnancy, but following oxcarbazepine MHD levels is advised. When an oxcarbazepine level is ordered in the clinical setting, the MHD concentration is always measured rather than the parent oxcarbazepine compound.

Levetiracetam

Levetiracetam is mostly eliminated through renal excretion, but about 25% is metabolized via extrahepatic hydrolysis. Levetiracetam levels decrease by 38–60% by the third trimester and clearance is found to increase by 243%, although significant interindividual variability is noted [52–54]. Limited case series [55] report no worsening of seizure frequency in patients on levetiracetam monotherapy. Other studies showed mixed results and no association between seizure worsening and levetiracetam level changes [53]. In another study, levetiracetam was used in combination with lamotrigine, rendering it unclear if changes in seizure frequency were due to lamotrigine [54]. There are no systematic studies currently available addressing the question of seizure frequency and levetiracetam levels, although levetiracetam level monitoring during pregnancy may be considered. Because the half-life of levetiracetam is relatively short, it may be especially important to compare levels at the same interval post dose if possible.

Topiramate

The major route of elimination for topiramate is renal excretion when used in monotherapy, and it has low binding to plasma proteins. Topiramate clearance is increased by 34–72% with a corresponding plasma level decrease of about 40%; however neither of the two small studies demonstrated a clear correlation between plasma topiramate level and seizure frequency [56,57]. The authors of both studies conclude that following topiramate levels during pregnancy might be of value.

Other AEDs

There are no systematic studies evaluating the pharmacokinetic effects of pregnancy on other newer AEDs, despite the fact that some of them have been available after approval for over 10–15 years. A single case study reports decrease in zonisamide serum concentrations, suggesting increased clearance at the end of the second trimester [58]. In general, for medications that are metabolized via glucuronidation and/or have high protein binding (e.g., tiagabine), a considerable effect of gestation is expected. The level of medications with high renal clearance (pregabalin, vigabatrin) is also expected to decrease substantially. It is reasonable to assume that AED levels will decrease during the gestational period, although substantial interindividual variations are possible. Therefore, it is justifiable to monitor AED levels regularly in all pregnant women with epilepsy, with monitoring of free (unbound) levels for those medications which are highly protein-bound.

Implications of AED pharmacokinetics after birth

In the postpartum period, reversal of the gestational physiologic changes is expected. These changes usually occur within weeks, but as early as within couple of days after birth. Decrease in AED clearance might lead to medication toxicity, if AED dosing is not decreased to pre-pregnancy levels in a timely manner. In general with all AEDs, postpartum taper should be planned. The rapidity of the postpartum pharmacokinetic changes are likely related to the major routes of metabolism, with some evidence that the reversal occurs most quickly for glucuronidation and renal excretion, while cytochrome P450 metabolism returns to baseline more slowly, up to a few months. Lamotrigine is the most-studied AED for postpartum pharmacokinetic changes. There are number of reports regarding symptomatic lamotrigine toxicity in the early postpartum period [41,59]. Another study [22] showed that using a planned empiric taper on postpartum days 3, 7, and 10 reduces the likelihood of maternal lamotrigine toxicity. The authors found this to be a clinically effective way to manage the postpartum alterations in lamotrigine metabolism, as obtaining a lamotrigine level in steady state with rapid physiologic changes is difficult and waiting for the results to make medication doses would likely be too late to avoid symptomatic toxicity. An approach involving either an empiric medication taper or for serial AED level monitoring for some AEDs, with gradual decrease of the dose until near pre-pregnancy levels are reached, is recommended for all AEDs that were increased during the pregnancy. If a woman has seizures that are sensitive to sleep deprivation, the clinician may choose to maintain the AED at a slightly higher dose than before conception until improved sleep patterns are reestablished [22].

Implications for management

The optimal management of AEDs in all pregnant women with epilepsy involves finding the delicate balance between minimizing possible teratogenic and developmental side effects on the fetus while maintaining seizure freedom. The same general principles should be considered in all women with epilepsy who are at childbearing age as about 50% of pregnancies are unplanned [14]. The understanding of how gestational physiologic changes alter the pharmacokinetic properties of certain AEDs is paramount in order to optimally manage women with epilepsy.

Ideally, pre-pregnancy management involves judicious planning time, when the aim is to achieve seizure control with monotherapy, or using the lowest number of medications possible. During this time, the lowest effective drug concentration needs to be determined. The effect of other medications on AED pharmacokinetics (i.e., oral contraceptives) needs to be taken into account and the individual target concentration reestablished after discontinuation of the contraceptive. Current recommendations are to obtain at least one, but preferably two, levels during stable seizure-free periods to establish the individualized pre-conceptional target concentration. Pre-gestational planning is shown to decrease seizure frequency during pregnancy [9].

It is difficult to predict the gestation-induced pharmacokinetic changes for most AEDs. A considerable effect of pregnancy on clearance is expected for AEDs metabolized via glucuronidation, as well as AEDs that are cleared renally and/or have high protein binding. Pregnancy-induced changes of cytochrome P450 hepatic metabolism also occur, but with less consistency. Substantial interindividual variations are possible with most AEDs. Following free levels of AEDs with high protein binding is recommended, as changes in free levels may be significantly different from total levels. There is convincing evidence for alterations in plasma concentration during pregnancy and monitoring is recommended for phenytoin, carbamazepine and lamotrigine, and more recently for levetiracetam and oxcarbazepine (Table 9.2). The evidence is insufficient to support or refute a change in phenobarbital, valproate, primidone, and ethosuximide, although lack of evidence should not discourage regular monitoring of levels and appropriate medication dose changes to maintain pre-pregnancy reference levels for these medications as well [32].

Physiologic changes after birth may lead to significant alteration in pharmacokinetics of some AEDs within weeks, in certain AEDs within days. Post-pregnancy taper guidelines are available for lamotrigine [22,60]. A planned postpartum taper schedule, with or without postpartum level monitoring, is recommended for all AEDs that were increased during the pregnancy.

Review of the case: A 32 year-old right-handed woman with history of complex partial seizures since age 17 was appropriately transitioned to lamotrigine at age 27 in preparation for her first pregnancy. Her pre-pregnancy levels were 11–12 µg/mL with excellent seizure control. It is unknown if these levels were obtained while she was taking oral contraceptives. During her first pregnancy, lamotrigine was increased 2.7 times higher than the pre-conception dose. Her pregnancy and postpartum period were complicated by lamotrigine toxicity, causing ataxia and unsteadiness for hours after taking the medication. It is not known whether lamotrigine toxicity was recognized and if levels were measured during or after pregnancy. It is also unclear what post-pregnancy taper was utilized. During her second pregnancy lamotrigine was increased only minimally, levels were maintained at 7.5–11.2 µg/mL, and she remained seizure-free. Empirical postpartum taper was done and she did not have any signs of toxicity. During her third pregnancy, a lower individualized lamotrigine target concentration was determined, and seizure freedom was maintained with levels of 6.3–7.9 µg/mL.

This case highlights the importance of (i) pregnancy planning with transition to an AED with abundant data supporting relatively low risk of structural and neurobehavioral teratogenicity, if possible; (ii) establishing the lowest effective dose (which might be lower than "official" therapeutic ranges) to further decrease teratogenic potential and developmental side effects on the fetus; (iii) close monitoring of AED levels during pregnancy and appropriate increase in dose considering the individual variability in concentration changes; (iv) recognition of clinical signs of medication toxicity; and (v) postpartum medication taper to avoid toxicity after pregnancyn.

💡 **Key summary points**

- Aim to avoid AEDs with a high teratogenic risk in all woman of childbearing potential.
- Plan for pregnancy, including in women not immediately trying to become pregnant.
- Aim for possible monotherapy and establish the lowest effective dose and concentration.

- Recheck levels after discontinuation of oral contraceptives and adjust dosage again if possible prior to conception.
- If available, use extended-release formulations of the AED to help accommodate increased clearance during pregnancy.
- Follow the total and free levels for AEDs that are highly protein-bound when available.
- Increase medication doses to reach pre-conception target levels.
- Plan for postpartum medication level taper.

References

1 Hauser WA, Annegers JF, Rocca WA. Descriptive epidemiology of epilepsy: contributions of population-based studies from Rochester, Minnesota. *Mayo Clin Proc* 1996;71:576–586.

2 Pack AM, Davis AR, Kritzer J, Yoon A, Camus A. Antiepileptic drugs: are women aware of interactions with oral contraceptives and potential teratogenicity? *Epilepsy Behav* 2009;14:640–644.

3 Meador KJ, Pennell PB, Harden CL *et al.* Pregnancy registries in epilepsy: a consensus statement on health outcomes. *Neurology* 2008;71:1109–1117.

4 Vajda FJ, Graham J, Roten A, Lander CM, O'Brien TJ, Eadie M. Teratogenicity of the newer antiepileptic drugs: the Australian experience. *J Clin Neurosci* 2012;19:57–59.

5 Morrow J, Russell A, Guthrie E *et al.* Malformation risks of antiepileptic drugs in pregnancy: a prospective study from the UK Epilepsy and Pregnancy Register. *J Neurol Neurosurg Psychiatry* 2006;77:193–198.

6 Meador KJ, Baker GA, Browning N *et al.* Cognitive function at 3 years of age after fetal exposure to antiepileptic drugs. *N Engl J Med* 2009;360:1597–1605.

7 Cohen MJ, Meador KJ, Browning N *et al.* Fetal antiepileptic drug exposure: motor, adaptive, and emotional/behavioral functioning at age 3 years. *Epilepsy Behav* 2011;22:240–246.

8 Nei M, Daly S, Liporace J. A maternal complex partial seizure in labor can affect fetal heart rate. *Neurology* 1998;51:904–906.

9 Sabers A. Influences on seizure activity in pregnant women with epilepsy. *Epilepsy Behav* 2009;15:230–234.

10 Gjerde IO, Strandjord RE, Ulstein M. The course of epilepsy during pregnancy: a study of 78 cases. *Acta Neurol Scand* 1988;78:198–205.

11 Holmes LB, Mittendorf R, Shen A, Smith CR, Hernandez-Diaz S. Fetal effects of anticonvulsant polytherapies: different risks from different drug combinations. *Arch Neurol* 2011;68:1275–1281.

12 Patsalos PN, Berry DJ, Bourgeois BF *et al.* Antiepileptic drugs: best practice guidelines for therapeutic drug monitoring: a position paper by the subcommission on therapeutic drug monitoring, ILAE Commission on Therapeutic Strategies. *Epilepsia* 2008;49:1239–1276.

13 Tomson T, Battino D, Bonizzoni E *et al.* Dose-dependent risk of malformations with antiepileptic drugs: an analysis of data from the EURAP epilepsy and pregnancy registry. *Lancet Neurol* 2011;10:609–617.

14 Finer LB, Henshaw SK. Disparities in rates of unintended pregnancy in the United States, 1994 and 2001. *Perspect Sex Reprod Health* 2006;38:90–96.

15 Reddy DS. Clinical pharmacokinetic interactions between antiepileptic drugs and hormonal contraceptives. *Expert Rev Clin Pharmacol* 2010;3:183–192.

16 Dutton C, Foldvary-Schaefer N. Contraception in women with epilepsy: pharmacokinetic interactions, contraceptive options, and management. *Int Rev Neurobiol* 2008;83:113–134.

17 Sabers A, Ohman I, Christensen J, Tomson T. Oral contraceptives reduce lamotrigine plasma levels. *Neurology* 2003;61:570–571.

18 Galimberti CA, Mazzucchelli I, Arbasino C, Canevini MP, Fattore C, Perucca E. Increased apparent oral clearance of valproic acid during intake of combined contraceptive steroids in women with epilepsy. *Epilepsia* 2006;47:1569–1572.

19 Sabers A, Tomson T. Managing antiepileptic drugs during pregnancy and lactation. *Curr Opin Neurol* 2009;22:157–161.

20 Pennell PB. Too complicated or so simple: AED type and AED dose matter for pregnancy. *Epilepsy Curr* 2012;12:1–3.

21 Pennell PB, Hovinga CA. Antiepileptic drug therapy in pregnancy I: gestation-induced effects on AED pharmacokinetics. *Int Rev Neurobiol* 2008;83:227–240.

22 Pennell PB, Peng L, Newport DJ *et al.* Lamotrigine in pregnancy: clearance, therapeutic drug monitoring, and seizure frequency. *Neurology* 2008;70:2130–2136.

23 Johannessen Landmark C, Johannessen SI, Tomson T. Host factors affecting antiepileptic drug delivery–pharmacokinetic variability. *Adv Drug Deliv Rev* 2012;64:896–910.

24 Ramsay RE, Strauss RG, Wilder BJ, Willmore LJ. Status epilepticus in pregnancy: effect of phenytoin malabsorption on seizure control. *Neurology* 1978;28:85–89.

25 Tomson T, Lindbom U, Ekqvist B, Sundqvist A. Epilepsy and pregnancy: a prospective study of seizure control in relation to free and total plasma concentrations of carbamazepine and phenytoin. *Epilepsia* 1994;35:122–130.

26 Yerby MS, Friel PN, McCormick K. Antiepileptic drug disposition during pregnancy. *Neurology* 1992;42:12–16.

27 Pennell PB. Antiepileptic drug pharmacokinetics during pregnancy and lactation. *Neurology* 2003;61:S35–S42.

28 Longo B, Forinash AB, Murphy JA. Levetiracetam use in pregnancy. *Ann Pharmacother* 2009;43:1692–1695.

29 Perucca E, Crema A. Plasma protein binding of drugs in pregnancy. *Clin Pharmacokinet* 1982;7:336–352.

30 Dickinson RG, Hooper WD, Wood B, Lander CM, Eadie MJ. The effect of pregnancy in humans on the pharmacokinetics of stable isotope labelled phenytoin. *Br J Clin Pharmacol* 1989;28:17–27.

31 Yerby MS, Friel PN, McCormick K *et al.* Pharmacokinetics of anticonvulsants in pregnancy: alterations in plasma protein binding. *Epilepsy Res* 1990;5:223–228.

32 Harden CL, Pennell PB, Koppel BS *et al.* Practice parameter update: management issues for women with epilepsy. Focus on pregnancy (an evidence-based review): vitamin K, folic acid, blood levels, and breastfeeding: report of the Quality Standards Subcommittee and Therapeutics and Technology Assessment Subcommittee of the American Academy of Neurology and American Epilepsy Society. *Neurology* 2009;73:142–149.

33 Battino D, Binelli S, Bossi L *et al.* Plasma concentrations of carbamazepine and carbamazepine 10,11-epoxide during pregnancy and after delivery. *Clin Pharmacokinet* 1985;10:279–284.

34 Bernus I, Hooper WD, Dickinson RG, Eadie MJ. Metabolism of carbamazepine and co-administered anticonvulsants during pregnancy. *Epilepsy Res* 1995;21:65–75.

35 Battino D, Binelli S, Bossi L *et al.* Changes in primidone/phenobarbitone ratio during pregnancy and the puerperium. *Clin Pharmacokinet* 1984;9:252–260.

36 Lander CM, Livingstone I, Tyrer JH, Eadie MJ. The clearance of anticonvulsant drugs in pregnancy. *Clin Exp Neurol* 1981;17:71–78.

37 Koerner M, Yerby M, Friel P, McCormick K. Valproic acid disposition and protein binding in pregnancy. *Ther Drug Monit* 1989;11:228–230.

38 Philbert A, Pedersen B, Dam M. Concentration of valproate during pregnancy, in the newborn and in breast milk. *Acta Neurol Scand* 1985;72:460–463.

39 Rating D, Nau H, Jäger-Roman E, *et al.* Teratogenic and pharmacokinetic studies of primidone during pregnancy and in the offspring of epileptic women. *Acta Paediatr Scand* 1982;71:301–311.

40 Kuhnz W, Koch S, Jakob S, Hartmann A, Helge H, Nau H. Ethosuximide in epileptic women during pregnancy and lactation period. Placental transfer, serum concentrations in nursed infants and clinical status. *Br J Clin Pharmacol* 1984;18:671–677.

41 Pennell PB, Newport DJ, Stowe ZN, Helmers SL, Montgomery JQ, Henry TR. The impact of pregnancy and childbirth on the metabolism of lamotrigine. *Neurology* 2004;62:292–295.

42 Tran TA, Leppik IE, Blesi K, Sathanandan ST, Remmel R. Lamotrigine clearance during pregnancy. *Neurology* 2002;59:251–255.

43 Fotopoulou C, Kretz R, Bauer S *et al.* Prospectively assessed changes in lamotrigine-concentration in women with epilepsy during pregnancy, lactation and the neonatal period. *Epilepsy Res* 2009;85:60–64.

44 Chen S, Beaton D, Nguyen N *et al.* Tissue-specific, inducible, and hormonal control of the human UDP-glucuronosyltransferase-1 (UGT1) locus. *J Biol Chem* 2005;280: 37547–37557.

45 Reimers A, Helde G, Brâthen G, Brodtkorb E. Lamotrigine and its N2 glucuronide during pregnancy: the significance of renal clearance and estradiol. *Epilepsy Res* 2011;94:198–205.

46 Tomson T, Luef G, Sabers A, Pittschieler S, Ohman I. Valproate effects on kinetics of lamotrigine in pregnancy and treatment with oral contraceptives. *Neurology* 2006;67:1297–1299.

47 Sabers A, Petrenaite V. Seizure frequency in pregnant women treated with lamotrigine monotherapy. *Epilepsia* 2009;50:2163–2166.

48 Christensen J, Sabers A, Sidenius P. Oxcarbazepine concentrations during pregnancy: a retrospective study in patients with epilepsy. *Neurology* 2006;67:1497–1499.

49 Mazzucchelli I, Onat FY, Ozkara C *et al.* Changes in the disposition of oxcarbazepine and its metabolites during pregnancy and the puerperium. *Epilepsia* 2006;47:504–509.

50 Wegner I, Edelbroek P, de Haan GJ, Lindhout D, Sander JW. Drug monitoring of lamotrigine and oxcarbazepine combination during pregnancy. *Epilepsia* 2010;51:2500–2502.

51 Petrenaite V, Sabers A, Hansen-Schwartz J. Seizure deterioration in women treated with oxcarbazepine during pregnancy. *Epilepsy Res* 2009;84:245–249.

52 Tomson T, Palm R, Kallen K *et al.* Pharmacokinetics of levetiracetam during pregnancy, delivery, in the neonatal period, and lactation. *Epilepsia* 2007;48:1111–1116.

53 Westin AA, Reimers A, Helde G, Nakken KO, Brodtkorb E. Serum concentration/dose ratio of levetiracetam before, during and after pregnancy. *Seizure* 2008;17:192–198.

54 Lopez-Fraile IP, Cid AO, Juste AO, Modrego PJ. Levetiracetam plasma level monitoring during pregnancy, delivery, and postpartum: clinical and outcome implications. *Epilepsy Behav* 2009;15:372–375.

55 Long L. Levetiracetam monotherapy during pregnancy: a case series. *Epilepsy Behav* 2003;4:447–448.

56 Ohman I, Sabers A, de Flon P, Luef G, Tomson T. Pharmacokinetics of topiramate during pregnancy. *Epilepsy Res* 2009;87:124–129.

57 Westin AA, Nakken KO, Johannessen SI, Reimers A, Lillestølen KM, Brodtkorb E. Serum concentration/dose ratio of topiramate during pregnancy. *Epilepsia* 2009;50:480–485.

58 Oles KS, Bell WL. Zonisamide concentrations during pregnancy. *Ann Pharmacother* 2008;42:1139–1141.

59 de Haan GJ, Edelbroek P, Segers J *et al*. Gestation-induced changes in lamotrigine pharmacokinetics: a monotherapy study. *Neurology* 2004;63:571–573.

60 Sabers A. Algorithm for lamotrigine dose adjustment before, during, and after pregnancy. *Acta Neurol Scand* 2012;126:e1–e4.

CHAPTER 10

Fetal and Maternal Risks with Seizures

Vilho K. Hiilesmaa and Kari A. Teramo

Department of Obstetrics and Gynecology, Helsinki University Central Hospital, Helsinki, Finland

> **Case history:** *The patient had been diagnosed with idiopathic epilepsy after three generalized tonic–clonic seizures since the age of 25. At the age of 28, she became pregnant for the first time. The last seizure had occurred 9 months before pregnancy. She regularly attended our outpatient clinic for pregnant women with epilepsy [1]. Her treatment was phenytoin 100mg daily, which was continued unchanged throughout pregnancy. Serum levels of the drug were below the usually recommended reference range, but the dose was not augmented because no seizures had occurred during pregnancy. Her pregnancy proceeded uneventfully and labor started spontaneously at term. A spiral electrode was attached to the fetal scalp for recording of fetal heart rate (FHR) when the cervix was 4cm dilated. About 1 hour later, the patient unexpectedly suffered a generalized tonic–clonic seizure, which lasted for 2.5min (see Figure 10.1). At the end of the seizure, she was treated with diazepam 10mg intravenously and 10mg intramuscularly. FHR decelerated below 120bpm, and the short-term variability decreased for more than 13min. After this there was a phase of tachycardia up to 165bpm with decreased short-term and long-term variablility. Half an hour after the beginning of the seizure a late deceleration was seen. A cesarean section was made 43min after the beginning of the seizure. A male infant weighed 3630g and received an Apgar score of 8 at the age of 1min. He recovered normally except for a slightly reduced muscular tone presumably due to diazepam. The concentration of phenytoin during delivery in maternal blood was only 0.9µg/mL (4µmol/L).*

General effects of seizures

Lactic acidosis

In adults with epilepsy, a generalized tonic–clonic seizure (GTCS) causes a marked lactic acidosis [2,3]. Orringer *et al.* [2] observed a mean pH of 7.14 immediately after a seizure in eight nonpregnant patients with epilepsy. During a seizure, lack of respiratory oxygen leads to anaerobic oxidation

---

Epilepsy in Women, First Edition. Edited by Cynthia L. Harden, Sanjeev V. Thomas and Torbjörn Tomson.

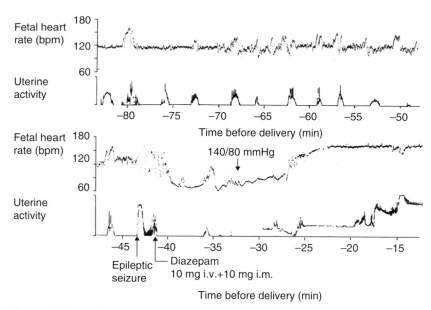

Figure 10.1 Fetal heart rate recorded via a scalp electrode and uterine activity before, during, and after a maternal clonic convulsive (grand mal) seizure during labor. (Reproduced with the permission of the authors and the publisher from Teramo K, Hiilesmaa V, Bardy A, Saarikoski S. Fetal heart rate during a maternal grand mal epileptic seizure. *J Perinat Med* 1979;7:3–6.)

which is followed by high concentrations of lactic acid due to intense muscular activity. Postictal apnea leads to hypoxia and can aggravate acidosis and delay the return to normal. After about 1 hour, spontaneous resolution of the acidosis has occurred and the mean pH returns to normal (7.38) [2].

Hypoxia and lactic acidosis presumably also develop in a pregnant woman with epilepsy as a result of GTCS and postictal apnea. These biochemical changes are transferred to the fetus because the placenta is fully and passively permeable to substances of low molecular weight such as blood gases and lactic acid.

We have reported on three women with epilepsy (including the case described above) in whom FHR was recorded via a scalp electrode before, during, and after a GTCS during labor [1,4]. The recordings showed marked changes in FHR during the following 45–60 min (Figures 10.1 and 10.2). These included bradycardia, lack of short-term and long-term variation, and late decelerations, followed by compensatory tachycardia. These changes are similar to those that occur during an acute episode of fetal hypoxia and acidosis.

Partial seizures can also produce changes in FHR suggesting hypoxia and acidosis. Sahoo and Klein [5] reported a mother who became hypoxic during a partial seizure during her seventh month of pregnancy. The FHR decelerated from 125 to 70 bpm for 2.5 min after the seizure. Nei *et al.* [6] reported a case of prolonged fetal bradycardia and prolonged uterine contractions for

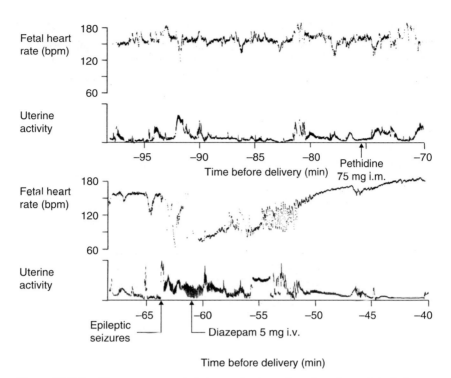

Figure 10.2 Fetal heart rate recorded via a scalp electrode and uterine activity before, during, and after a maternal clonic convulsive (grand mal) seizure during labor. (Reproduced with the permission of the authors and the publisher from Hiilesmaa VK, Bardy A, Teramo K. Obstetric outcome in women with epilepsy. *Am J Obstet Gynecol* 1985;152:499–504.)

4 min immediately after a partial seizure during labor at term. The intrauterine pressure measurement peaked abnormally high (above 100 mmHg). The maternal and fetal outcome was good in both of these case reports [5,6].

Circulatory changes

A GTCS causes marked cardiovascular changes in both humans [7] and experimental animals [8]. The blood flow to the brain increases markedly. Much of the arterial blood flow is directed to the musculature. Very little is known about uterine and placental blood flow during a maternal seizure. It is not known whether fetal hypoxia is produced by decreased placental blood flow due to a redistribution of maternal blood flow or to an increase in uterine tone during a seizure. Another possibility might be postictal maternal apnea and acidosis transferred to the fetus [1].

Uterine contractions

A GTCS during pregnancy or labor can increase uterine contractions during and after a seizure [1] (see Figures 10.1 and 10.2). The same has been observed also for partial seizures occurring during pregnancy or labor [5,6].

The increased uterine tone and contractions can temporarily reduce arterial blood flow to the placenta, and at least partially explain the decelerations observed in FHR [1,4–6]. Premature rupture of fetal membranes or preterm labor have not been associated with seizure-induced uterine contractions.

Trauma to the uterus

It is conceivable that placental abruption could occur during a convulsive epileptic seizure, particularly if the patient falls. Vaginal bleeding in late pregnancy was found increased in a recent study on women with epilepsy, but it was not due to placental abruption [9]. It has been shown in non-epileptic women that a fall during late pregnancy can cause blunt trauma to the uterus, which can lead to fetomaternal hemorrhage [10,11]. Even a minor injury can lead to a clinically significant fetomaternal hemorrhage resulting in severe fetal anemia [12]. One of our patients with an intrauterine FHR registration during labor fell from the bed to the floor, but this did not hurt her or the fetus [1]. Although significant physical trauma to the uterus after a GTCS has not been reported in the literature, it is possible that a large uterus could be injured if a woman with epilepsy falls and hurts herself during a seizure.

Seizures and fetal malformations

Current reports on the risk of seizures causing malformations

There are a few prospective clinical studies in which patients were recruited in early pregnancy and in which the occurrence of seizures during the first trimester was recorded [13–15]. In these studies, multivariate analyses did not show independent associations between GTCS during the first trimester and an increased risk of major congenital malformations.

Evaluating teratogenic effects of seizures

Moderate association between seizures and malformations cannot be excluded based on the negative results in the above-mentioned studies. First, only 6–8% of all pregnant women with epilepsy have a GTCS during the first trimester [13,15]. Second, the "first trimester" has not been offi-cially defined; it is usually considered as comprising the postmenstrual weeks 2–13, whereas the sensitive period of organogenesis (during which most major malformations develop) only consists of weeks 5–8. Given that the seizures occur at random times throughout the first trimester, it can be calculated that only about 2–3% of all women with epilepsy have seizures that occur in the short period of organogenesis, whereas about 70–80% of the fetuses of women with epilepsy are continuously exposed to maternal antiepileptic medication. Therefore, much larger studies would be required to verify or exclude teratogenic potential of seizures than what is needed for evaluating the effects of commonly used antiepileptic drugs (AEDs).

Limitations in register-based research

Although most large register-based publications on epilepsy and pregnancy contain adequate information on drug exposure and have access to the diagnosis of epilepsy, they often lack data on the occurrence and timing of seizures because that information was not originally required to be recorded in the databases on which these registers are based [9,16].

Seizures and spontaneous abortions

Results in current reports

While some studies have found an increased rate of spontaneous abortion among women with epilepsy [17,18], others suggest that the rate is similar to that in general populations [19]. In the large EURAP study on seizures during pregnancy, none of the 133 spontaneous abortions occurred in close proximity to a seizure or status epilepticus [14]. It is also noteworthy that 74% of the spontaneous abortions in the EURAP study occurred in women who did not have seizures during pregnancy.

Definition of spontaneous abortion

The exact number of spontaneous abortions is difficult to estimate, and much more so in retrospective studies. An early miscarriage may pass unnoticed as a slightly delayed abundant menstruation if a pregnancy test is not done [20]. In the general population, about 15–20% of pregnancies diagnosed by pregnancy test or ultrasonography end in spontaneous abortion. The earlier a pregnancy test is made, the more pregnancies are diagnosed and the greater will be the proportion that ends in miscarriage. It may be speculated that women with epilepsy would try to verify their pregnancy earlier than women who do not have specific risk factors. Without a rigorous definition of spontaneous abortion its incidence is rendered uncertain. In light of current knowledge, there is no evidence that epileptic seizures could notably increase the risk of spontaneous abortions.

Seizures and common obstetric complications

Occurrence of pregnancy complications in women with epilepsy

Increased numbers of pregnancy and birth complications in women with epilepsy have been observed in several studies. However, no consistent pattern emerges. A complication that is found increased in one study is lacking in another. A slight excess of virtually all common obstetric complications among women with epilepsy have been reported in the literature [20]. These include preterm labor [9,21], growth restriction [22,23], preeclampsia [9,18,24], nonproteinuric gestational hypertension [9,18,25], intrauterine infections [18], anemia [18,21], increased uterine bleeding [9,18,24,26], and low Apgar scores [22,27]. There are studies which did not find increase in any pregnancy complications in women with epilepsy [4].

Role of seizures in pregnancy complications

None of the above-mentioned reports suggested an association between seizures and pregnancy complications. A recent evidence-based review concluded that there is no substantially increased risk of common pregnancy complications among women with epilepsy, although a slight increase in most of these cannot be reliably excluded [28]. Another study based on national health registries suggests a slightly increased rate of preterm births and low birthweight due to seizures in women with epilepsy [29]. However, in this study there were no direct data on the occurrence of seizures. The authors defined women with seizures during pregnancy as those who were hospitalized or treated in the emergency department for epilepsy during pregnancy.

While maternal seizures during pregnancy can be clinically evaluated, the concomitant long-term effects may be hidden and difficult to register and assess. Seizures in pregnancy usually occur outside hospital, and the patient has already recovered when she attends the healthcare system after a seizure. Only when there is evidence that the rates of certain pregnancy complications are indeed increased, and when there are reliable data on seizures during pregnancy, will it be possible to meaningfully study the eventual impact of seizures in pregnancy.

Seizures and maternal deaths

Thirty years ago, we found 29 case reports with status epilepticus during pregnancy in the medical literature between the years 1910 and 1978 [30]. These included nine maternal deaths. The incidence of these events during this time period is unknown. In the developed countries today, a maternal death is very rare. However, an investigation into maternal deaths in the UK showed that the odds for maternal death were about 10 times higher for women with epilepsy than for the general population. The case histories suggested that these deaths were often due to seizures following poor compliance or discontinuing of antiepileptic medication [31]. Furthermore, a recent report found that the risk of sudden unexpected death in subjects with epilepsy is more than 20 times higher than that in the general population [32]. Despite the increased relative risk, the absolute risk of maternal death remains very small. For instance, none of the recent large studies of pregnant women with epilepsy and pregnancy reports maternal deaths even in cases of status epilepticus [9,13,14,16,27]. However, all maternal deaths may not always be reported to the registers.

Comparing historical and current reports, it is obvious that, during the few last decades, there has been a drastic improvement in both the neurological and obstetric care of patients. Today, even severe forms of epilepsy, including those with a risk of status epilepticus, do not carry a significant risk of maternal death, provided adequate care is available.

Seizures and stillbirths

A stillbirth is defined as a fetal death after 22 completed weeks of pregnancy. Perinatal deaths comprise stillbirths and neonatal deaths during the first week of life. In our review of the old literature up to the 1970s, we found three isolated case reports on a fetal death associated with a single maternal seizure [30]. There were also 29 reported cases of status epilepticus during pregnancy, with at least 14 fetal deaths *in utero* or shortly after birth [30]. However, the incidence of these events at that time is not known because no epidemiologic studies had been made.

Between 1970 and 1990, several epidemiologic studies suggested a 1.2-fold to threefold increase in perinatal deaths in pregnancies of women with epilepsy [20]. In the recent EURAP study there were 30 (1.5%) stillbirths among 1956 pregnancies in women with epilepsy [14]. This is about twofold to threefold as compared with the recent figures in the developed world [33]. Of these 30 stillbirths in the EURAP study, one was due to maternal status epilepticus. Seizures occurred in half of the remaining 29 pregnancies, but no temporal association between seizures and stillbirths was observed [14]. There are also recent series in which the rate of stillbirths was similar to that in the background populations [9,18].

Based on the literature, it can be concluded that the number of stillbirths among women with epilepsy is slightly increased (1.2–3 times). The reasons for this remain unclear. An isolated GTCS or partial seizure does not carry notable immediate risk for intrauterine death but status epilepticus is more dangerous in this respect [14]. However, hidden and delayed fetal effects of seizures could contribute to the number of stillbirths but so far there is no evidence thereof. Furthermore, among women with epilepsy other factors are possibly associated with an increased risk of stillbirth, such as low social class and adverse effects of severe burden of medication which, inevitably, are associated with more severe epilepsy [31]. Separating the effects of seizures from those due to other factors will obviously be difficult.

Seizures and childbirth (i.e., labor, delivery and early puerperium)

Probability of seizures during childbirth

The reports agree that labor and delivery carry an elevated risk of epileptic seizures [14,20,34]. The incidence of seizures during this period has been estimated to be nine times greater than that during pregnancy in general [34]. During childbirth, 3–4% of women with epilepsy have seizures of which about half are GTCS [14,34]. Mental and physical stress, often associated with lack of sleep during vaginal childbirth, obviously increase the risk of having seizures.

In the EURAP study, the probability of seizures occurring during labor or delivery was fivefold if there had been seizures earlier during pregnancy [14]. On the other hand, this study found that 14 of 60 patients with seizures during childbirth had been seizure-free throughout the entire pregnancy. Furthermore, five women with only nonconvulsive seizures during pregnancy unexpectedly developed convulsive seizures during childbirth [14]. Thus, it is possible to predict to a certain extent whether seizure(s) will occur in the upcoming labor and delivery. The increased risk of seizures continues for 1–2 days after delivery [34].

Effects of seizures during childbirth

As described in detail at the beginning of this chapter, a GTCS is followed by lactic acidosis, redistribution of blood circulation (possibly including reduced flow to uterus), and increased uterine activity as evidenced by fetal cardiotocographic monitoring during labor (see Figures 10.1 and 10.2) [1,4]. Similar findings have also been reported during and after partial seizures [5,6].

The effects of a single seizure usually subside within an hour [1,2]. The infants born after a maternal seizure are usually in good condition and receive normal Apgar scores [1,4–6]. Delivery is often by cesarean section due to postictal inability of the mother to further cooperate during labor, but also because of suspected fetal distress. A healthy fetus seems to tolerate a maternal seizure during labor. However, if there is underlying fetal compromise, such as growth restriction, anemia, or chronic hypoxia (e.g., due to maternal diabetes), a maternal GTCS could be fatal for the fetus.

Seizure at childbirth: eclampsia, epilepsy or something else?

Patients with eclampsia typically have preeclampsia (pregnancy-induced hypertension and proteinuria) days or weeks prior to the seizure. Furthermore, eclampsia is often preceded by typical prodromal symptoms, such as nausea, vomiting, headaches, and visual disturbances. In these cases there is no problem in making the correct diagnosis.

Likewise, when a patient with a history of epilepsy does not show signs of preeclampsia and develops a seizure during childbirth, the diagnosis obviously is epilepsy. When the patient has her first-ever seizure during childbirth unrelated to preeclampsia and without a history of epilepsy, the underlying cause may not be immediately evident. Then other possibilities, such as sinus thrombosis, brain tumor, aneurysm of the brain, or medication- or drug-related seizures, should also be considered. This is discussed in more detail in Chapter 7.

Late child effects of maternal seizures during pregnancy

Clinical studies
In a study from the UK, multiple regression analysis showed that both valproate exposure and five or more tonic–clonic seizures in pregnancy were significantly associated with a lower verbal IQ in children despite adjusting for other confounding factors. The authors warn that the results need to be interpreted with caution given their retrospective nature [31].

In a prospective study of children of women with epilepsy, no association was found between occurrence of seizures and intelligence in the offspring [35,36]. However the limited size of the study population reduces its power to show or exclude such effects with reasonable confidence.

Experimental studies
Experimental studies on the effects of seizures without AED treatment during pregnancy on later development of the offspring are contradictory. In a small study in rhesus monkeys with focal motor seizures and phenytoin treatment during pregnancy, motor and social impairment of the offspring correlated directly with the phenytoin dose during the third trimester of pregnancy but not with maternal seizure frequency during gestation [37]. In a rat model, induced epileptic seizures during pregnancy resulted in placental infarctions and deficits in motor coordination of the offspring [38]. However, in a similar rat model, seizures during pregnancy had no adverse effects on neurobehavioral maturation of the offspring [39]. In both of these studies a healthy foster dam was used to take care of the rat pups. Clearly, more studies, both experimental and clinical, are needed to evaluate the effects of maternal seizures on later development of the offspring.

Implications for management

Since there is evidence that GTCSs and extensive partial seizures can have marked and potentially ominous effects on the expectant mother and her fetus [1,2,4–6], these types of seizures should be avoided throughout pregnancy and at the time of childbirth. In practice, this means that AED medication has to be used in the majority of patients, from pre-pregnancy planning until puerperium. It is important to encourage patients to continue antiepileptic treatment during pregnancy as needed despite the fear of fetal malformations [31].

A fall in a pregnant woman can result in blunt trauma to a large uterus [11]. The same presumably applies to a woman who falls during an epileptic seizure. Some clinics, including ours, recommend that the pregnant patient visit her obstetric clinic immediately after a GTCS to ensure maternal and fetal well-being.

The risk of seizures during labor, delivery, and the immediate postpartum period is increased among women with epilepsy [14,34]. About 3–4% have seizures during childbirth, of which half are GTCSs. It is possible, up to a certain degree, to predict the occurrence of seizures during childbirth, but the absence of a GTCS during pregnancy does not guarantee freedom from this type of seizure during the upcoming childbirth [14].

Augmentation of the antiepileptic treatment at 33–36 weeks should be considered in patients who have seizures during pregnancy to provide additional protection during the childbirth. Administration of AEDs may be neglected during the childbirth. It has been shown that the lowest concentrations of AEDs throughout the entire pregnancy may occur during labor and delivery [40]. The personnel at the delivery unit and the patient herself should ensure that there will be no delays or omissions of her medication. It is also to be recommended that the patient bring her AEDs to the hospital when the labor starts. Obstetric units may not have all the newest or seldom used AEDs immediately available at all times. Also, it has to be remembered that the increased risk of seizures continues for 1–2 days after delivery, which should be taken into account in the postnatal care [34].

The delivery of women with epilepsy should preferably take place in a hospital with sufficient preparedness to handle eventual seizures during labor and delivery and other specific problems.

> **Review of the case:** The case history presented here illustrates clinically important issues related to childbirth of a woman with epilepsy. This patient's risk of having a seizure during childbirth was estimated as low because she had had no seizures during pregnancy. Therefore, her medication was considered adequate despite the low serum levels. An additional point was to reduce fetal exposure to a minimum. A lesson here is

that absence of seizures during pregnancy does not guarantee absence of seizures during childbirth. The marked changes in FHR after the seizure suggesting fetal hypoxia and acidosis are of general importance since the same probably occurs throughout pregnancy. Another noteworthy finding is the very low serum concentration of the AED at delivery. The patient assured the staff that she had taken her medication regularly. In retrospect, it could have been beneficial to increase her dose for the last few weeks of pregnancy to ensure adequate AED medication during the childbirth. The rapid and complete recovery of the newborn suggests that a healthy fetus is well able to tolerate a maternal GTCS during childbirth.

 Key summary points

1. A GTCS and postictal apnea cause hypoxia and lactic acidosis, which are transferred to the fetus through the placenta.

2. Seizures induce contractions and may reduce uterine and placental blood circulation.

3. Seizures can cause a blunt trauma to a large uterus if the patient falls.

4. After a GTCS an obstetric check-up is recommended.

5. No association between seizures and malformations or pregnancy complications has been observed so far but the power of current studies is insufficient to prove or exclude such harmful effects.

6. During labor, delivery and 1–2 days thereafter, 3–4% of women with epilepsy have seizure(s). The obstetric unit should be capable of handling seizures during childbirth.

7. Good control of seizures is even more important during pregnancy than it is at other times of life.

References

1 Teramo K, Hiilesmaa V, Bardy A, Saarikoski S. Fetal heart rate during a maternal grand mal epileptic seizure. *J Perinat Med* 1979;7:3–6.

2 Orringer CE, Eustace JC, Wunsch CD, Gardner LB. Natural history of lactic acidosis after grand-mal seizures. A model for the study of an anion-gap acidosis not associated with hyperkalemia. *N Engl J Med* 1977;297:796–799.

3 Lipka K, Bülow HH. Lactic acidosis following convulsions. *Acta Anaesthesiol Scand* 2003;47:616–618.

4 Hiilesmaa VK, Bardy A, Teramo K. Obstetric outcome in women with epilepsy. *Am J Obstet Gynecol* 1985;152:499–504.

5 Sahoo S, Klein P. Maternal complex partial seizure associated with fetal distress. *Arch Neurol* 2005;62:1304–1305.

6 Nei M, Daly S, Liporace J. A maternal complex partial seizure in labor can affect fetal heart rate. *Neurology* 1998;51:904–906.

7 Meyer JS, Gotoh F. Cerebral metabolism during epileptic seizures in man. *Trans Am Neurol Assoc* 1965;90:23–29.

8 Plum F, Posner JB, Troy B. Cerebral metabolic and circulatory responses to induced convulsions in animals. *Arch Neurol* 1968;18:1–13.

9 Borthen I, Eide MG, Veiby G, Daltveit AK, Gilhus NE. Complications during pregnancy in women with epilepsy: population-based cohort study. *BJOG* 2009;116: 1736–1742.

10 Goodwin TM, Breen MT. Pregnancy outcome and fetomaternal hemorrhage after noncatastrophic trauma. *Am J Obstet Gynecol* 1990;162:665–671.

11 Pearlman MD, Tintinalli JE, Lorenz RP. A prospective controlled study of outcome after trauma during pregnancy. *Am J Obstet Gynecol* 1990;162:1502–1507.

12 Tarvonen M, Ulander VM, Süvari L, Teramo K. [Minor trauma during pregnancy can cause severe fetomaternal hemorrhage.] *Duodecim* 2011;127:1727–1731.

13 Kaaja E, Kaaja R, Hiilesmaa V. Major malformations in offspring of women with epilepsy. *Neurology* 2003;60:575–579.

14 EURAP Study Group. Seizure control and treatment in pregnancy: observations from the EURAP epilepsy pregnancy registry. *Neurology* 2006;66:354–360.

15 Tomson T, Battino D, Bonizzoni E *et al.* Dose-dependent risk of malformations with antiepileptic drugs: an analysis of data from the EURAP epilepsy and pregnancy registry. *Lancet Neurol* 2011;10:609–617.

16 Artama M, Auvinen A, Raudaskoski T, Isojärvi I, Isojärvi J. Antiepileptic drug use of women with epilepsy and congenital malformations in offspring. *Neurology* 2005;64:1874–1878.

17 Schupf N, Ottman R. Reproduction among individuals with idiopathic/cryptogenic epilepsy: risk factors for spontaneous abortion. *Epilepsia* 1997;38:824–829.

18 Thomas SV, Sindhu K, Ajaykumar B, Sulekha Devi PB, Sujamol J. Maternal and obstetric outcome of women with epilepsy. *Seizure* 2009;18:163–166.

19 Annegers JF, Baumgartner KB, Hauser WA, Kurland LT. Epilepsy, antiepileptic drugs, and the risk of spontaneous abortion. *Epilepsia* 1988;29:451–458.

20 Hiilesmaa VK. Pregnancy and birth in women with epilepsy. *Neurology* 1992;42 (Suppl 5):8–11.

21 Svigos JM. Epilepsy and pregnancy. *Aust NZ J Obstet Gynaecol* 1984;24:182–185.

22 Viinikainen K, Heinonen S, Eriksson K, Kälviäinen R. Community-based, prospective, controlled study of obstetric and neonatal outcome of 179 pregnancies in women with epilepsy. *Epilepsia* 2006;47:186–192.

23 Al Bunyan M, Abo-Talib Z. Outcome of pregnancies in epileptic women: a study in Saudi Arabia. *Seizure* 1999;8:26–29.

24 Borthen I, Eide MG, Daltveit AK, Gilhus NE. Obstetric outcome in women with epilepsy: a hospital-based, retrospective study. *BJOG* 2011;118:956–965.

25 Richmond JR, Krishnamoorthy P, Andermann E, Benjamin A. Epilepsy and pregnancy: an obstetric perspective. *Am J Obstet Gynecol* 2004;190:371–379.

26 Mawer G, Briggs M, Baker GA *et al.* Pregnancy with epilepsy: obstetric and neonatal outcome of a controlled study. *Seizure* 2010;19:112–119.

27 Borthen I, Eide MG, Daltveit AK, Gilhus NE. Delivery outcome of women with epilepsy: a population-based cohort study. *BJOG* 2010;117:1537–1543.

28 Harden CL, Hopp J, Ting TY *et al.* Practice parameter update: management issues for women with epilepsy. Focus on pregnancy (an evidence-based review): obstetrical complications and change in seizure frequency. *Neurology* 2009;73:126–132.

29 Chen YH, Chiou HY, Lin HC, Lin HL. Affect of seizures during gestation on pregnancy outcomes in women with epilepsy. *Arch Neurol* 2009;66:979–984.

30 Teramo K, Hiilesmaa VK. Pregnancy and fetal complications in epileptic pregnancies. In: Janz D, Dam M, Bossi L, Helge H, Richens A, Schmidt D (eds) *Epilepsy, Pregnancy, and the Child.* New York: Raven Press, 1982: 53–59.

31 Adab N, Kini U, Vinten J *et al.* The longer term outcome of children born to mothers with epilepsy. *J Neurol Neurosurg Psychiatry* 2004;75:1575–1583.

32 Shorvon S, Tomson T. Sudden unexpected death in epilepsy. *Lancet* 2011;378: 2028–2038.

33 Stanton C, Lawn JE, Rahman H, Wilczynska-Ketende K, Hill K. Stillbirth rates: delivering estimates in 190 countries. *Lancet* 2006;367:1487–1494.

34 Bardy AH. Incidence of seizures during pregnancy, labor and puerperium in epileptic women: a prospective study. *Acta Neurol Scand* 1987;75:356–360.

35 Gaily E, Kantola-Sorsa E, Granstrom ML. Intelligence of children of epileptic mothers. *J Pediatr* 1988;113:677–684.

36 Gaily E, Kantola-Sorsa E, Hiilesmaa V *et al.* Normal intelligence in children with prenatal exposure to carbamazepine. *Neurology* 2004;62:28–32.

37 Phillips NK, Lockard JS. A gestational monkey model: effects of phenytoin versus seizures on neonatal outcome. *Epilepsia* 1985;26:697–703.

38 Lima DC, Gurgel de Vale T, Arganãraz GA *et al.* Behavioral evaluation of adult rats exposed in utero to maternal epileptic seizures. *Epilepsy Behav* 2010;18:45–49.

39 Raffo E, Pereira de Vascocelos A, Boehrer A, Desor D, Nehlig A. Neurobehavioral maturation of offspring from epileptic dams: study in the rat lithium–pilocarpine model. *Exp Neurol* 2009;219:414–423.

40 Bardy AH, Hiilesmaa VK, Teramo KA. Serum phenytoin during pregnancy, labor and puerperium. *Acta Neurol Scand* 1987;75:374–375.

CHAPTER 11

Obstetrical Outcome and Complications of Pregnancy

Ingrid Borthen[1] *and Nils Erik Gilhus*[2]

[1]Department of Obstetrics of Neurology, Department of Clinical Medicine, University of Bergen, Haukeland University Hospital, Bergen, Norway

[2]Department of Clinical Medicine, University of Bergen, and Department of Neurology, Haukeland University Hospital, Bergen, Norway

---

Case history: *This 25-year-old woman was consulting her general practitioner. She was diagnosed with juvenile myoclonic epilepsy at the age of 16. She was using valproate and has been seizure-free for the last 5 years. Now she was planning to become pregnant. She wanted to stop the medication due to its teratogenic effects. She was referred to a neurologist who advised her to change medication to lamotrigine, starting with 100mg twice daily, as her epilepsy was liable to recurrence without medication. After 3 months with the new medication, she came back for a new consultation. She had no seizures and felt comfortable with her medication. Her doctor advised her to start folic acid 4mg/day to reduce the risk of malformation. She became pregnant after 4 months and was referred to the antenatal clinic in the obstetrical department for follow-up. She reduced the dose of folic acid to 0.4mg at 12 weeks and at the same time had an early ultrasound scan and another scan at 18 weeks. The fetus had no detectable malformations and the mother was in good shape. The obstetric department was following her pregnancy at monthly intervals. In week 34, her blood pressure was increasing to 170/100mmHg and she was hospitalized. After 3 days, she had proteins in her urine, first mild and then increasing to 7.5g per 24 hours. Her blood pressure was increasing to 180/120mmHg, and she was delivered by cesarean section in week 35. The baby's weight was 2440g and Apgar score 8 after 1 min and 9 after 5 min.*

Introduction

Epilepsy is a common neurological disease in pregnancy with an estimated prevalence of 0.3–0.7% [1–3]. Studies have reported reduced fertility in women with epilepsy [4]. However, women with epilepsy have lower marriage rates, and fertility among married women with epilepsy seems to

---

Epilepsy in Women, First Edition. Edited by Cynthia L. Harden, Sanjeev V. Thomas and Torbjörn Tomson.

be comparable to married women in the general population [4,5]. Most women with epilepsy will have normal pregnancies with healthy babies. However, there is an increased risk of complications compared with the general population [3,6]. Seizures can be more severe and frequent, and there is an increased risk of malformations in the offspring [7]. It is important to be aware of this increased risk as proper management may minimize the risk for both mother and fetus.

Pre-conception dialogue

Women with epilepsy should plan their pregnancies and this should be emphasized by doctors treating young females. Use of medication is important to keep them seizure-free during pregnancy. However, antiepileptic drugs (AEDs) may cause major congenital malformations [8] and lead to adverse effects on cognitive development [9]. Several studies have demonstrated an increased risk of major congenital malformations [10], adverse cognitive effects [11], and decreased intelligence with the use of valproate during pregnancy [12]. There seems to be a lower risk with the use of monotherapy [10] and the AED dose seems to be an important risk factor of major congenital malformations [10]. The use of AEDs has to be balanced against the need to keep the mother seizure-free. A consultation before conception should focus on need for medication, type of medication, use of monotherapy, and lowest dose possible.

Folate use

AEDs such as valproate, carbamazepine, phenobarbital, phenytoin, and primidone alter folic acid metabolism, and folic acid blood levels decrease with increasing plasma levels of these AEDs [13]. The use of folic acid supplementation is generally accepted as important prior to conception and during pregnancy in women on AEDs, with the aim of reducing the risk of neural tube defects [14]. However, data on the benefits of folic acid supplementation come from studies of women without epilepsy but who are at high risk of having a child with neural tube defects [15]. Studies aimed at assessing the effects in fetuses with AED exposure have failed to show a convincing protective effect against major congenital malformations [16]. This may be due to limitations in study design, but could also be due to an inability of folic acid to overcome AED-related teratogenic mechanisms or because the doses prescribed to women on AEDs are inadequate [17]. Nevertheless, folic acid supplementation is recommended for women with epilepsy, as it is for all women of childbearing age, starting supplementary intake when they stop contraception [14]. The recommended dose of folic acid is debated and there are insufficient data to provide clear advice. Wald *et al.* [18] systematically reviewed ingested folate dose, resulting serum concentrations, and influence on neural tube defects. They concluded that 5 mg/day of folate is necessary to render 85% protection. However, this study was performed on patients without epilepsy and the results cannot be transferred to patients with epilepsy without further investigation. Studies of folate use in women with epilepsy lack convincing results. The American Academy of Neurology recommends at least 0.4 mg/day [19], while the UK NICE guidelines recommend all women on AEDs be given 5 mg of folic acid daily before any possibility of pregnancy [14]. Additional studies from the epilepsy registries will be needed to advise correctly on the dosing of folic acid. Until convincing results are published, a dose of 4–5 mg daily to women using carbamazepine, phenobarbital, phenytoin, primidone, and valproate should be recommended, starting 3 months before conception and continuing until 12 weeks past conception. The dose after 12 weeks should be 0.4 mg. All users of other AEDs should be given a dose of at least 0.4 mg folic acid daily.

Complications of pregnancy

Women with epilepsy are often considered at high risk in pregnancy. Two studies on women treated with the older-generation AEDs have reported increased risks of bleeding in pregnancy, preeclampsia, and preterm birth [20,21], but this has not been replicated in other studies [3,22,23]. It has been discussed whether differences in AED use or in the included epilepsy population are responsible for these differences [24]. One of the studies reported an increased risk of gestational hypertension in women with epilepsy [3]. This finding was supported by three recent studies reporting a higher incidence of preeclampsia [odds ratio (OR) 1.5–2.2] and gestational hypertension (OR 1.4) in women with epilepsy treated with AEDs [6,25,26].

Preeclampsia results from an imbalance between factors produced by the placenta and maternal adaptation to them [27]. Factors such as oxidative stress, circulating placenta-derived proteins, immunological defects, and genetic variance may all be important [28]. Recently, a three-stage model of preeclampsia has been suggested, only the last stage being the manifest clinical illness [27]. AEDs such as carbamazepine and lamotrigine may lower serum calcium levels and increase parathyroid hormone [29], as well as decreasing serum folic acid, all factors associated with occurrence of preeclampsia and hypertension [30,31].

Vaginal bleeding in pregnancy has been listed as a possible complication for women with epilepsy. Two previous studies could not detect any such increased risk [22,32], in contrast to two recent studies where a significantly increased risk was identified both early (OR 6.4) and late (OR 1.9) in pregnancy in women with epilepsy using AEDs [6,26]. Vaginal bleeding occurred most often with carbamazepine and lamotrigine treatment [26,33]. AED-induced folic acid deficiency and alteration in the metabolism of vitamin K-dependent blood clotting factors have been suggested as causes of vaginal bleeding in late pregnancy [34]. Carbamazepine can lower folic acid levels; lamotrigine can also reduce folic acid levels as the drug has a slight inhibitory effect on dihydrofolate reductase.

Postpartum hemorrhage, defined as bleeding of more than 500 mL [35], has been evaluated in only a few studies of women with epilepsy, with no increased risk observed [2,4,23]. In contrast, two recent studies found an increased rate of bleeding among women using AEDs during pregnancy (OR 1.5) [33,36], especially in those using oxcarbazepine and valproate. Uterine atony may account for the increased incidence. As the rate of cesarean delivery was high in the women with epilepsy, the increased bleeding may also reflect the high cesarean rate in these women. The same mechanisms that lead to the increased risk of bleeding in pregnancy most probably also contribute to the increased bleeding after birth.

An increased risk for preterm delivery has been observed in women with epilepsy using AEDs [20,37] and use of carbamazepine was associated with the highest risk [33]. However, other studies have not been able to replicate any difference in preterm labor [3,25].

Delivery

In studies from the last decade, women with epilepsy have been at increased risk of being induced for labor, even though epilepsy was not an indication for the induction. According to guidelines, induction of labor should be evaluated on an individual basis [14,38].

A major issue in obstetrical practice is that cesarean section rates are rising worldwide, and also for women with epilepsy. In a recent study, women with epilepsy using AEDs had a higher risk of being delivered by caesarean section than the reference women without epilepsy (OR 1.6) [37]. The study was not able to identify any pregnancy complications explaining the increased caesarean delivery rate. Most chronic disorders increase the likelihood of caesarean delivery [39]. Epilepsy represents a significant disorder, but is not by itself an indication for caesarean delivery. Studies have observed similar rates of vacuum and forceps deliveries in women with and without epilepsy [3,26,37], reflecting similar complication rates in both groups.

Obstetrical outcome

The offspring of women with epilepsy not using AEDs have the same rate of major congenital malformations as offspring of women without epilepsy [33]. There are no differences in Apgar score and birthweight [33]. However, children of women with epilepsy using AEDs have an increased risk of intrauterine growth restriction. Causative factors could be the epilepsy, exposure to AEDs, seizures, genetic factors, any underlying condition causing the epilepsy, and environmental factors including lifestyle. The growth restriction was most pronounced in children exposed to carbamazepine and oxcarbazepine. Head circumference in AED-exposed children was also reduced, as well as body length [40]. This is in accordance with newer registry studies [33,41]. A study from Sweden estimated the effect on head growth of exposure *in utero* to the new AEDs lamotrigine and gabapentin, and the old AEDs phenytoin, clonazepam, carbamazepine, and valproate [41]. Carbamazepine had the strongest effect, whereas phenytoin, clonazepam, lamotrigine, and gabapentin had no such effects. Polytherapy increased the risk of microcephaly compared with children not exposed to AEDs and in the same weight group (OR 2.85). Low birthweight (<2500 g) and small head circumference occurred significantly more frequently in AED-exposed infants of mothers with epilepsy, and was most pronounced in children exposed to carbamazepine and polytherapy in a Norwegian study [33].

Implications for management

Women with epilepsy should have a consultation before conception to discuss medications and possible complications in pregnancy. Monotherapy is preferable and in the lowest dose possible. Valproate should be avoided. However, it is important to emphasize that the risk for malformations is low. Folate supplementation should be started at least 3 months before pregnancy for all women using AEDs. As there is an increased risk of malformations with use of medications, women with epilepsy using AEDs should be referred to an ultrasound screening in week 11–12. The pregnancy should be followed by her general practitioner, obstetricians, and neurologists together. The fetus should be monitored by ultrasound to evaluate growth. Blood pressure measurements and urine proteins every fourth week is important to detect preeclampsia. Delivery should take place in a specialized hospital as some women will have seizures during delivery. Whether to pursue vaginal versus caesarean delivery should be based solely on obstetrical considerations.

> **Review of the case:** *Our patient demonstrates problems in pregnancy seen with increased frequency when on medications with AEDs. Carbamazepine and lamotrigine are often preferred for young females because of their acceptable side-effect profile, including a low risk of major malformations, when used in low doses. However, there is a slightly increased risk of the pregnancy complications preeclampsia, bleeding in pregnancy, and preterm birth. These complications might influence the health of the children in later life.*

 Key summary points

1. Pre-conceptional consultation by neurologist and obstetrician.

2. Folic acid from 3 months before conception: 4–5 mg/day with use of enzyme-inducing drugs or 0.4 mg/day with other drugs. Reduce the dose of 0.4 mg at week 12.

3. Blood pressure and urine examination every fourth week or on obstetrical considerations.

4. Serum level of drugs used every fourth week or on neurological considerations.

5. Ultrasound screening week 11–12.

6. Ultrasound screening week 18.

7. Follow-up by neurologist and obstetrician every 4–8 weeks.

8. Delivery based on obstetrical considerations in specialized units

References

1 Hauser WA, Annegers JF, Rocca WA. Descriptive epidemiology of epilepsy: contributions of population-based studies from Rochester, Minnesota. *Mayo Clin Proc* 1996;71:576–586.

2 Hiilesmaa VK, Bardy A, Teramo K. Obstetric outcome in women with epilepsy. *Am J Obstet Gynecol* 1985;152:499–504.

3 Richmond JR, Krishnamoorthy P, Andermann E, Benjamin A. Epilepsy and pregnancy: an obstetric perspective. *Am J Obstet Gynecol* 2004;190:371–379.

4 Olafsson E, Hallgrimsson JT, Hauser WA, Ludvigsson P, Gudmundsson G. Pregnancies of women with epilepsy: a population-based study in Iceland. *Epilepsia* 1998;39: 887–892.

5 Artama M, Isojärvi JI, Raitanen J, Auvinen A. Birth rate among patients with epilepsy: a nationwide population-based cohort study in Finland. *Am J Epidemiol* 2004;159:1057–1063.

6 Borthen I, Eide MG, Veiby G, Daltveit AK, Gilhus NE. Complications during pregnancy in women with epilepsy: population-based cohort study. *BJOG* 2009;116: 1736–1742.

7 Battino D, Tomson T. Management of epilepsy during pregnancy. *Drugs* 2007;67: 2727–2746.

8 Meador K, Reynolds MW, Crean S, Fahrbach K, Probst C. Pregnancy outcomes in women with epilepsy: a systematic review and meta-analysis of published pregnancy registries and cohorts. *Epilepsy Res* 2008;81:1–13.

9 Meador KJ, Baker GA, Browning N *et al.* Cognitive function at 3 years of age after fetal exposure to antiepileptic drugs. *N Engl J Med* 2009;360:1597–1605.

10 Morrow J, Russell A, Guthrie E *et al.* Malformation risks of antiepileptic drugs in pregnancy: a prospective study from the UK Epilepsy and Pregnancy Register. *J Neurol Neurosurg Psychiatry* 2006;77:193–198.

11 Bromley RL, Baker GA, Meador KJ. Cognitive abilities and behaviour of children exposed to antiepileptic drugs in utero. *Curr Opin Neurol* 2009;22:162–166.

12 Eriksson K, Viinikainen K, Mönkkönen A *et al.* Children exposed to valproate in utero: population based evaluation of risks and confounding factors for long-term neurocognitive development. *Epilepsy Res* 2005;65:189–200.

13 Dansky LV, Rosenblatt DS, Andermann E. Mechanisms of teratogenesis: folic acid and antiepileptic therapy. *Neurology* 1992;42(4 Suppl 5):32–42.

14 National Institute for Health and Clinical Excellence. *Epilepsies: The Diagnosis and Management of the Epilepsies in Adults and Children in Primary and Secondary Care.* Clinical Guideline 20. Available at www.nice.org.uk/guidance/CG20.

15 MRC Vitamin Study Research Group. Prevention of neural tube defects: results of the Medical Research Council Vitamin Study. *Lancet* 1991;338:131–137.

16 Morrow JI, Hunt SJ, Russell AJ *et al.* Folic acid use and major congenital malformations in offspring of women with epilepsy: a prospective study from the UK Epilepsy and Pregnancy Register. *J Neurol Neurosurg Psychiatry* 2009;80:506–511.

17 Pack AM. Therapy insight: clinical management of pregnant women with epilepsy. *Nat Clin Pract Neurol* 2006;2:190–200.

18 Wald NJ, Law MR, Morris JK, Wald DS. Quantifying the effect of folic acid. *Lancet* 2001;358:2069–2073.

19 Harden CL, Pennell PB, Koppel BS *et al.* Practice parameter update: management issues for women with epilepsy. Focus on pregnancy (an evidence-based review): vitamin K, folic acid, blood levels, and breastfeeding: report of the Quality Standards Subcommittee and Therapeutics and Technology Assessment Subcommittee of the American Academy of Neurology and American Epilepsy Society. *Neurology* 2009;73:142–149.

20 Bjerkedal T, Bahna SL. The course and outcome of pregnancy in women with epilepsy. *Acta Obstet Gynecol Scand* 1973;52:245–248.

21 Yerby M, Koepsell T, Daling J. Pregnancy complications and outcomes in a cohort of women with epilepsy. *Epilepsia* 1985;26:631–635.

22 Viinikainen K, Heinonen S, Eriksson K, Kälviäinen R. Community-based, prospective, controlled study of obstetric and neonatal outcome of 179 pregnancies in women with epilepsy. *Epilepsia* 2006;47:186–192.

23 Katz O, Levy A, Wiznitzer A, Sheiner E. Pregnancy and perinatal outcome in epileptic women: a population-based study. *J Matern Fetal Neonatal Med* 2006;19:21–25.

24 Kaplan PW, Norwitz ER, Ben-Menachem E *et al.* Obstetric risks for women with epilepsy during pregnancy. *Epilepsy Behav* 2007;11:283–291.

25 Thomas SV, Sindhu K, Ajaykumar B, Sulekha Devi PB, Sujamol J. Maternal and obstetric outcome of women with epilepsy. *Seizure* 2009;18:163–166.

26 Borthen I, Eide MG, Daltveit AK, Gilhus NE. Obstetric outcome in women with epilepsy: a hospital-based, retrospective study. *BJOG* 2011;118:956–965.

27 Redman CW, Sargent IL. Immunology of pre-eclampsia. *Am J Reprod Immunol* 2010;63:534–543.

28 Staff AC, Dechend R, Pijnenborg R. Learning from the placenta: acute atherosis and vascular remodeling in preeclampsia. Novel aspects for atherosclerosis and future cardiovascular health. *Hypertension* 2010;56:1026–1034.

29 von Wegerer J, Hesslinger B, Berger M, Walden J. A calcium antagonistic effect of the new antiepileptic drug lamotrigine. *Eur Neuropsychopharmacol* 1997;7:77–81.

30 Hofmeyr GJ, Lawrie TA, Atallah AN, Duley L. Calcium supplementation during pregnancy for preventing hypertensive disorders and related problems. *Cochrane Database Syst Rev* 2010;(8):CD001059.

31 Timmermans S, Jaddoe VW, Silva LM *et al.* Folic acid is positively associated with uteroplacental vascular resistance: the Generation R Study. *Nutr Metab Cardiovasc Dis* 2011;21:54–61.

32 Hiilesmaa VK. Pregnancy and birth in women with epilepsy. *Neurology* 1992;42 (4 Suppl 5):8–11.

33 Veiby G, Daltveit AK, Engelsen BA, Gilhus NE. Pregnancy, delivery, and outcome for the child in maternal epilepsy. *Epilepsia* 2009;50:2130–2139.

34 Donaldson JO. Neurological disorders. In: de Swiet M (ed.) *Medical Disorders in Obstetric Practice.* Oxford: Blackwell Science, 2002: 486–489.

35 Cunningham FG, MacDonald PC, Gant NF, Gilstrap LC, Hankins GD, Clark SL (eds) Obstetrical hemorrhage. In: *Williams Obstetrics.* New York: Appelton & Lange, 1997: 745–783.

36 Pilo C, Wide K, Winbladh B. Pregnancy, delivery, and neonatal complications after treatment with antiepileptic drugs. *Acta Obstet Gynecol Scand* 2006;85:643–646.

37 Borthen I, Eide MG, Daltveit AK, Gilhus NE. Delivery outcome of women with epilepsy: a population-based cohort study. *BJOG* 2010;117:1537–1543.

38 Taubøll E, Gjerstad L, Henriksen T, Husby H. [Women and epilepsy.] *Tidsskr Nor Laegeforen* 2003;123:1691–1694.

39 Linton A, Peterson MR. Effect of preexisting chronic disease on primary cesarean delivery rates by race for births in U.S. military hospitals, 1999–2002. *Birth* 2004;31:165–175.

40 Hvas CL, Henriksen TB, Ostergaard JR, Dam M. Epilepsy and pregnancy: effect of antiepileptic drugs and lifestyle on birthweight. *BJOG* 2000;107:896–902.

41 Almgren M, Kallen B, Lavebratt C. Population based study of antiepileptic drug exposure in utero: influence on head circumference in newborns. *Seizure* 2009;18:672–675.

CHAPTER 12

Mechanisms of Teratogenic Effects of AEDs

Lynsey E. Bruce, Ana M. Palacios, Bogdan J. Wlodarczyk and Richard H. Finnell

Dell Pediatric Research Institute, Department of Nutritional Sciences, University of Texas at Austin, Austin, Texas, USA

Background and important detail

Despite the widely reported adverse effects and overall impact of antiepileptic drug (AED) use in pregnant patients, little is known about the mechanisms of teratogenicity for these drugs. There is a nearly 50-year history documenting the teratogenic potential of AEDs in humans, making them a singularly important class of pharmaceutical compounds that are well-established human teratogens. Yet much of the data available on the teratogenic effects of AEDs and their potential targets has been derived from studies in animal models. There is a critical lack of understanding of how these drugs impact not only the patients themselves, but also the developing embryo. The extent to which specific AEDs cross the placenta is important in determining the total concentration of drug that reaches the developing embryo. AED dosage also appears to be a factor in the teratogenic risk. A combination of these factors has informed our ideas about how AEDs may disrupt normal development in susceptible embryos. The goal of this chapter is to address some of the more widely studied mechanisms of teratogenicity for AEDs, and how these mechanisms may influence the management of pregnant epileptic women. We discuss four of the proposed hypotheses that have received the greatest attention, and the AEDs that have been implicated as owing their teratogenicity to one or more of these mechanisms. This is followed by a discussion of the implications for management of epilepsy in pregnant women, based on these primary hypotheses.

Epoxidation

Biotransformation of certain AEDs via epoxidation is believed to yield reactive intermediary compounds that may be responsible for the teratogenicity of some of the AEDs. Epoxides are generated during the metabolism of aromatic compounds when a catalytic reaction with oxygen creates an ether ring within the parent molecule. The resulting triangular structure is highly strained, which may result in a molecule that is more reactive and potentially mutagenic.

The cytochrome P450 (CYP) superfamily, which is highly involved in drug metabolism and bioactivation, are the enzymes largely responsible for epoxide generation. CYPs account for about 75% of drug metabolism [1], and it has been shown that some AED intermediate molecules target substrates for CYP activity. The induction or inhibition of CYPs may be a major source of observed adverse drug reactions. In the case of drug polytherapy, altered CYP activity due to one drug may affect the metabolism and clearance of the second therapeutic compound. For example, felbamate inhibits CYP2C19, which causes an increase in the plasma concentration of phenytoin (PHT) [2,3]. This accumulation of PHT may result in the toxicity threshold being exceeded, thus causing a variety of adverse effects in the patient as well as in the developing embryo that would not have been observed if either of the two drugs was administered in monotherapy.

CYPs catalyze a monooxygenase reaction that results in the insertion of an oxygen atom into the substrate. In the case of AEDs, epoxide intermediates may result in toxic compounds that, if not rapidly eliminated, have the potential to interact with and bind to fetal macromolecules. Under normal circumstances, the enzyme epoxide hydrolase functions to detoxify epoxides to *trans*-dihydrodiols that are conjugated and eliminated from the body. However, deficiencies in this enzyme may result in accumulation of epoxide intermediates in patients taking AEDs that are aromatic in structure, which may lead to teratogenic effects.

Carbamazepine is a CYP inducer and therefore it increases the clearance of other drugs that do not interfere with its activity. Coincidentally, early studies on the teratogenic mechanisms of carbamazepine metabolism found that CYPs are also involved in the metabolism of the drug through the formation of a stable carbamazepine-10,11-epoxide intermediate (Figure 12.1) [4]. This epoxide intermediate has been hypothesized to be primarily responsible for the teratogenicity associated with the parent compound. This was supported by studies in pregnant mice which, when treated with carbamazepine-10,11-epoxide, resulted in a significant increase in the number of observed fetal malformations [5].

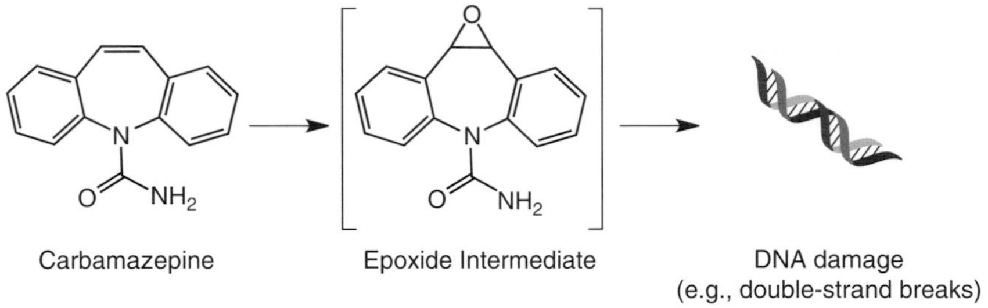

Carbamazepine   Epoxide Intermediate   DNA damage
                                                     (e.g., double-strand breaks)

Figure 12.1 Epoxidation by carbamazepine. Carbamazepine is metabolized into an epoxide intermediate during its bioactivation. Epoxides are highly reactive molecules that may interact with critical cellular biomolecules such as DNA. These interactions may cause DNA damage, such as double-strand breaks. Accumulation of these harmful intermediates during drug metabolism is believed to contribute to the teratogenicity of antiepileptic drugs.

PHT, a CYP inducer, is metabolized in a way that results in an epoxide intermediate, specifically an arene oxide that is produced during its bioactivation by CYP2C9 and CYP2C19 [6,7]. Arene oxides are highly reactive molecules that are capable of covalently binding nucleophilic sites found in embryonic macromolecules, should the rate of their bioactivation exceed the ability for the organism to detoxify [6,8,9]. This binding may interfere with normal embryonic development by initiating mutagenesis of critical regions of DNA, altering the structure of essential proteins in such a way as to inhibit their activity, or leading to the destruction of lipid membranes. For this reason, these epoxide intermediates have been impli-cated as potential mediators for mutations and malformations observed in children exposed *in utero* to AEDs.

Oxidative stress

Oxidative stress is a potential mechanism of the teratogenicity of a few AEDs, including PHT, valproic acid (VPA), and phenobarbital. It is well known that the generation of reactive oxygen species (ROS) due to oxidative stress conditions may damage DNA, proteins, and lipids. ROS, as their name implies, are molecules containing oxygen that are highly reactive due to unpaired valence shell electrons on the oxygen atom. ROS such as hydrogen peroxide and oxygen ions are generated during normal cellular metabolism, and play important roles in homeostasis and normal cellular signaling. CYPs, due to their role as catalysts for the oxidation of organic compounds, are critical contributors to ROS genera-tion during cellular oxidative stress. AED treatment induces environ-mental stress conditions during pregnancy, leading to an increase in the

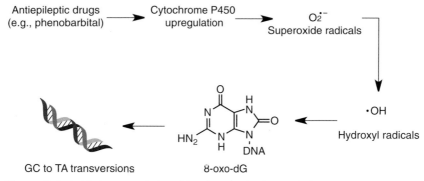

Figure 12.2 Oxidative stress induced by phenobarbital. Metabolism of antiepileptic drugs such as phenobarbital may alter cytochrome P450 activity. This results in the generation of superoxide radicals, which then leads to an accumulation of reactive hydroxyl radicals. These harmful reactive oxygen species are normally handled by endogenous cellular antioxidant mechanisms, but over-production of these free radical intermediates may overwhelm these systems. If left unchecked, these free radicals have the potential to react with DNA and form 8-oxo-2′-deoxyguanosine (8-oxo-dG). 8-oxo-dG results in GC to TA transversions within DNA, causing potentially mutagenic and irreversible damage.

formation of ROS in the developing embryo. AED polytherapy in particular has been implicated as a significant contributor to oxidative stress in the cell. Generation of these ROS during embryonic development negatively impacts normal cellular function by altering important proteins and nucleic acids involved in proliferation, differentiation, and apoptosis. This leads to disruption of normal embryo/fetal development, resulting in long-term defects.

As previously mentioned, epoxide intermediates have been implicated in the teratogenicity of PHT. However, an alternative theory, based on both *in vivo* and *in vitro* evidence, involves the oxidative stress model of teratogenicity. PHT is co-oxidized to free radical intermediates that may result in oxidative stress, lipid peroxidation, and/or covalent binding to essential nucleic acids [10,11]. As a result, PHT induces oxidation of DNA through similar means as phenobarbital. In fact, DNA oxidation following PHT treatment has been shown to induce homologous recombination as a result of double-strand DNA breaks in Chinese hamster ovary (CHO) cell lines [12]. Elevated numbers of double-strand DNA breaks are known to cause deleterious genetic changes, which may underlie the teratogenicity of AEDs that are capable of inducing oxidative stress in the developing embryo.

Phenobarbital has been shown to upregulate CYPs and potentiate the generation of superoxide radicals (Figure 12.2) [13]. Superoxides yield an accumulation of hydroxyl radicals that contribute to the formation of 8-oxo-2′-deoxyguanosine (8-oxo-dG). 8-oxo-dG is a major product of DNA oxidation that results in transversion of GC to TA within the genome, and its concentration within the cell is often used as a marker of oxidative stress. 8-oxo-dG transversions in critical developmentally regulated genes may lead to the generation of aberrant proteins, causing a variety of adverse effects that have the potential to disrupt normal development.

VPA is a known inhibitor of CYP activity. One of the many proposed mechanisms for VPA's teratogenicity may be partly due to CYP-mediated changes in its metabolism, which leads to the accumulation of toxic intermediates [14]. Both *in vivo* and *in vitro* studies on the mechanism of VPA teratogenicity has revealed that it does induce a state of oxidative stress in the developing embryo. VPA was shown to produce an increase in the formation of ROS in embryonic stem cells and post-implantation embryos, and this increase in ROS was shown to inhibit cardiomyocyte differentiation [15,16]. Furthermore, the increase in ROS was attenuated by catalase supplementation in post-implantation embryos [16], indicating that at least a portion of VPA's mechanism of teratogenicity may be due to oxidative stress. This also suggests that CYPs are not the only generators of oxidative stress conditions secondary to AED therapy.

Altered folate metabolism

Folate metabolism has long been considered an essential process for normal embryonic development. Folic acid is known to promote cellular growth and red blood cell maturation, and is required for DNA synthesis and repair and DNA methylation to regulate gene expression. Folic acid deficiency is associated with reduced growth, anemia, and neural tube defects in the developing embryo [17]. Folic acid deficiency is also associated with elevated levels of homocysteine in patients taking certain AEDs, and supplementation with folic acid was found to restore serum folic acid concentrations and lower homocysteine levels [18,19].

Results of multiple epidemiological studies have led to recommendations for women of childbearing age to take folic acid supplementation as a means to prevent selected birth defects, especially neural tube defects, congenital heart defects, and oral clefts [20,21]. Because of the importance of folate metabolism during embryonic development, the teratogenic nature of some AEDs has been attributed to their ability to alter the folate metabolic pathway. An AED-induced folic acid deficiency may explain why some AEDs taken during pregnancy result in congenital defects.

Most studies indicate that VPA does not directly reduce folate levels [22,23]. However, it has been suggested that teratogenic doses of VPA may indirectly alter folate metabolism by increasing levels of tetrahydrofolate and decreasing 5-formyl- and 10-formyl-tetrahydrofolate molecules.

A closely related, yet nonteratogenic structural analog of VPA that also has antiepileptic activity does not adversely affect folate metabolism [23,24]. Interestingly, VPA treatment did not result in increased homocysteine levels in patients [25].

PHT also appears to be involved in folate metabolism (Figure 12.3). An early study on PHT found that this drug acts as a folate antagonist, thereby inducing folic acid deficiency [26]. A 90% decrease in serum and red blood cell folate levels has been observed in patients receiving PHT or carbamazepine [27]. Patients taking phenobarbital or primidone often have low levels of serum folate as well [22,28]. Reduction in folate levels has significant implications for pregnant women, as pregnancy results in an increased overall demand for folates. If these demands are not met, this may adversely affect the developing embryo, resulting in abnormal growth and development.

A study on lamotrigine found that supplementation with folic acid rescued the cleft palate phenotype in mice, therefore negating the teratogenic effects of this drug [29]. However, a study on the effects of lamotrigine in human patients found that it had no effect on serum or red blood cell folate levels in patients who were on the drug in the short or long term [30]. These results are part of the reason why it is so difficult to identify a single causative mechanism for the teratogenicity of AEDs.

Histone deacetylases

Gene expression is largely regulated by the acetylation and deacetylation of the proteins known as histones, around which DNA is wrapped. Histones have a cumulative positive charge due to a large number of lysine and arginine amino acids. This positive charge allows histones to interact closely with the phosphate backbone of DNA generating a highly condensed chromatin structure. However, the highly condensed nature of chromatin makes it difficult for transcriptional machinery to access portions of DNA. Therefore, there is a need for proteins that can reduce the positive charge on histones, usually via acetylation, thus reducing DNA–histone interactions and loosening the chromatin structure, allowing access to genes that are transcriptionally active. Reversal of this process requires deacetylation of histone tails, thereby restoring the affinity of the DNA and histones.

Histone deacetylases (HDACs) are responsible for the deacetylation of lysine residues on histone tails, which leads to chromatin condensation and transcriptional repression. Besides interacting directly with histones, HDACs are also known to interact with some transcription factors and coregulators. Because of their importance, disturbances in HDAC activity can result in the disruption of normal cellular functions, thus affecting the

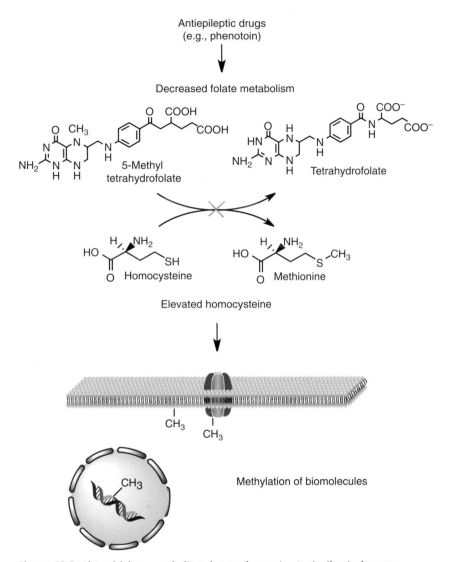

Figure 12.3 Altered folate metabolism due to phenytoin. Antiepileptic drug use
has been suggested to impact the metabolism of folic acid. Phenytoin, for instance,
has been shown to decrease folate metabolism. Normally, homocysteine is converted
to methionine during folate metabolism. This decrease in folate metabolism leads
to an accumulation of homocysteine, which is responsible for the methylation of DNA/
histones, lipids, and proteins. Methylation causes alterations in gene expression,
enzymatic activity, and membrane structure. These changes are thought to contribute
to the clinical defects (anemia, reduced fetal growth, neural tube defects) observed in
patients with folic acid deficiency, and to the teratogenesis of the drug.

highly orchestrated and rapid proliferation of cells in a growing embryo.
Inhibition of HDAC activity may inhibit cell growth and induce terminal
differentiation and/or apoptosis, which can disrupt the pattern of embryonic

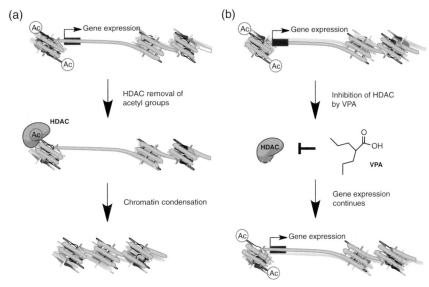

Figure 12.4 Histone deacetylase inhibition by valproic acid. (a) Acetylation of histones causes relaxation of chromatin, allowing genes within this region to be expressed. When the gene no longer needs to be expressed, histone deacetylases (HDACs) remove the acetyl groups from histone tails, allowing chromatin to recondense. (b) Valproic acid (VPA) has been implicated as an inhibitor of HDACs, a potential mechanism of teratogenicity that would lead to prolonged gene expression with potentially debilitating effects.

development. For this reason, the proposed HDAC model for the teratogenicity of AEDs has been among the most provocative and promising in recent years. Phiel *et al.* [31] and Gottlicher *et al.* [32] have suggested that HDACs may be targets for VPA, and that inhibition of HDAC activity by VPA may be responsible for its observed teratogenic effects (Figure 12.4). In fact, there is a direct correlation between somite hyperacetylation and axial abnormalities in embryos exposed to VPA [33]. A study performed *in vitro* confirmed inhibition of HDACs and induced histone hyperacetylation with VPA treatment in human HeLa cell lines [34]. These authors also found that two of the newer generation AEDs, topiramate and 2-pyrrolidinone-*N*-butyric acid, the major metabolite of levetiracetam, had the same inhibitory effects on HDACs.

Implications for management

The management of epilepsy during pregnancy remains a challenge in light of the potential teratogenic effects of antiepileptic medications. VPA is one of the most efficient wide-spectrum agents in the treatment of epilepsy. However, epidemiological studies have consistently demonstrated that it represents one of the highest risks of teratogenicity for the human embryo in both monotherapy and polytherapy exposures. This is supported by findings that the possible mechanism of VPA teratogenicity may be multifactorial, including oxidative stress, altered folate metabolism, and the potential inhibitory role of VPA in the function of HDACs, as evidenced in the previous section. It is worth mentioning that VPA teratogenicity in humans appears to be dose-dependent, and is thought to yield detrimental effects in postnatal neurocognitive and behavioral development of individuals who were exposed *in utero* to this drug.

The popularity of VPA usage in women of reproductive age has declined over the past few years. The use of first-generation AEDs has slowly been replaced by newer compounds, which are believed to be inherently safer and reduce the risk of teratogenicity in the embryo. However, presently available human pregnancy data on these newer drugs are still scarce. A recent study reported that the most commonly used antiseizure agent in both the USA and the UK is lamotrigine [35]. However, these investigators also found that levetiracetam, topiramate, oxcarbazepine, and zonisamide are more frequently used in the USA, while carbamazepine and VPA are more frequently used in the UK. Therefore, more information is needed on the mechanisms of these drugs and their effects in order to establish a safer treatment regimen for use in women of reproductive age.

In general, polytherapy regimens appear to exhibit an increased risk of teratogenicity in the exposed embryo when compared with monotherapy approaches, especially when VPA is one of the compounds [36]. Meador *et al.* [35] reported that pregnant women were less likely to be under a polytherapy regimen than nonpregnant women in the USA and the UK. Additionally, the most frequently prescribed combination of two AEDs in women of reproductive age in the USA comprised lamotrigine and levetiracetam, while in the UK it was carbamazepine and levetiracetam, providing further evidence of the decreasing trends for use of VPA and other older AEDs during pregnancy. More recently, Morrow *et al.* [36] found that coadministration of lamotrigine with VPA can decrease the teratogenicity of VPA. Anderson *et al.* [37] demonstrated using nonpregnant volunteers that lamotrigine increased the clearance of VPA. It has been proposed that lamotrigine alters VPA glucuronidation, causing increased clearance of VPA and thus reducing its plasma level and therefore lowering its teratogenicity. It is also possible that lamotrigine may, to a certain extent, be altering the formation of teratogenic VPA metabolites. Since this is the first study documenting this phenomenon, further research is needed to confirm this novel finding. Confirmation that lamotrigine decreases VPA teratogenicity will be of high clinical importance, since VPA remains one of the most effective and widely used of all AEDs.

Treatment of epilepsy during pregnancy remains a challenging clinical task. When a polytherapy regimen is considered, particular caution should be observed due to the increased risk for congenital malformations to occur. Pharmacological interactions between AEDs are not well studied in terms of their teratogenesis, although they are thought to be associated with an increased risk of birth defects in the developing embryo. In polytherapy, the likelihood of teratogenic effects usually increases. This may be due to different drugs having a shared mechanism of teratogenicity and is simply an additive effect.

 Key summary points

- Despite being used as therapeutic drugs for a long time, the mechanisms underlying the teratogenicity of AEDs are not well understood.
- The best-documented mechanisms for AED teratogenicity are induction of oxidative stress, formation of toxic epoxide intermediates, altered folate metabolism, and inhibition of HDACs.
- Some AEDs can exert their teratogenic potential via more than one mechanism.
- Very little is known about the mechanism of teratogenicity of the second-generation AEDs.
- AED polytherapy has been linked with higher risk of teratogenic outcome.
- In order to prevent the congenital malformations induced by AEDs, it is necessary to determine how they exert their teratogenic potential.

References

1 Guengerich FP. Cytochrome p450 and chemical toxicology. *Chem Res Toxicol* 2008;21: 70–83.
2 Glue P, Banfield CR, Perhach JL, Mather GG, Racha JK, Levy RH. Pharmacokinetic interactions with felbamate. In vitro–in vivo correlation. *Clin Pharmacokinet* 1997;33: 214–224.
3 Fuerst RH, Graves NM, Leppik IE, Brundage RC, Holmes GB, Remmel RP. Felbamate increases phenytoin but decreases carbamazepine concentrations. *Epilepsia* 1988;29: 488–491.
4 Lindhout D, Hoppener RJ, Meinardi H. Teratogenicity of antiepileptic drug combinations with special emphasis on epoxidation (of carbamazepine). *Epilepsia* 1984;25:77–83.
5 Bennett GD, Amore BM, Finnell RH *et al*. Teratogenicity of carbamazepine-10, 11-epoxide and oxcarbazepine in the SWV mouse. *J Pharmacol Exp Ther* 1996;279: 1237–1242.
6 Martz F, Failinger C III, Blake DA. Phenytoin teratogenesis: correlation between embryopathic effect and covalent binding of putative arene oxide metabolite in gestational tissue. *J Pharmacol Exp Ther* 1977;203:231–239.
7 Lum JT, Wells PG. Pharmacological studies on the potentiation of phenytoin teratogenicity by acetaminophen. *Teratology* 1986;33:53–72.

8 Jerina DM, Daly JW. Arene oxides: a new aspect of drug metabolism. *Science* 1974;185:573–582.

9 Strickler SM, Dansky LV, Miller MA, Seni MH, Andermann E, Spielberg SP. Genetic predisposition to phenytoin-induced birth defects. *Lancet* 1985;ii:746–749.

10 Wells PG, Vo HP. Effects of the tumor promoter 12-*O*-tetradecanoylphorbol-13-acetate on phenytoin-induced embryopathy in mice. *Toxicol Appl Pharmacol* 1989; 97:398–405.

11 Kubow S, Wells PG. In vitro bioactivation of phenytoin to a reactive free radical intermediate by prostaglandin synthetase, horseradish peroxidase, and thyroid peroxidase. *Mol Pharmacol* 1989;35:504–511.

12 Winn LM, Kim PM, Nickoloff JA. Oxidative stress-induced homologous recombination as a novel mechanism for phenytoin-initiated toxicity. *J Pharmacol Exp Ther* 2003;306:523–527.

13 Waxman DJ, Azaroff L. Phenobarbital induction of cytochrome P-450 gene expression. *Biochem J* 1992;281:577–592.

14 Sankar R. Teratogenicity of antiepileptic drugs: role of drug metabolism and pharmacogenomics. *Acta Neurol Scand* 2007;116:65–71.

15 Na L, Wartenberg M, Nau H, Hescheler J, Sauer H. Anticonvulsant valproic acid inhibits cardiomyocyte differentiation of embryonic stem cells by increasing intracellular levels of reactive oxygen species. *Birth Defects Res A Clin Mol Teratol* 2003;67:174–180.

16 Tung EW, Winn L. Valproic acid increases formation of reactive oxygen species and induces apoptosis in postimplantation embryos: a role for oxidative stress in valproic acid-induced neural tube defects. *Mol Pharmacol* 2011;80:979–987.

17 Morrell MJ. Folic acid and epilepsy. *Epilepsy Currents* 2002;2:31–34.

18 Ono H, Sakamoto A, Eguchi T *et al.* Plasma total homocysteine concentrations in epileptic patients taking anticonvulsants. *Metabolism* 1997;46:959–962.

19 Schwaninger M, Ringleb P, Winter R *et al.* Elevated plasma concentrations of homocysteine in antiepileptic drug treatment. *Epilepsia* 1999;40:345–350.

20 Botto LD, Mulinare J, Erickson JD. Do multivitamin or folic acid supplements reduce the risk for congenital heart defects? Evidence and gaps. *Am J Med Genet A* 2003; 121:95–101.

21 MRC Vitamin Study Research Group. Prevention of neural tube defects: results of the Medical Research Council Vitamin Study. *Lancet* 1991;338:131–137.

22 Kishi T, Fujita N, Eguchi T, Ueda K. Mechanism for reduction of serum folate by antiepileptic drugs during prolonged therapy. *J Neurol Sci* 1997;145:109–112.

23 Apeland T, Mansoor MA, Strandjord RE. Antiepileptic drugs as independent predictors of plasma total homocysteine levels. *Epilepsy Res* 2001;47:27–35.

24 Wegner C, Nau H. Alteration of embryonic folate metabolism by valproic acid during organogenesis: implications for mechanism of teratogenesis. *Neurology* 1992;42(4 Suppl 5):17–24.

25 Apeland T, Mansoor MA, Strandjord RE, Kristensen O. Homocysteine concentrations and methionine loading in patients on antiepileptic drugs. *Acta Neurol Scand* 2000;101:217–223.

26 Matsui MS, Rozovski SJ. Drug–nutrient interaction. *Clin Ther* 1982;4:423–440.

27 Ogawa Y, Kaneko S, Otani K, Fukushima Y. Serum folic acid levels in epileptic mothers and their relationship to congenital malformations. *Epilepsy Res* 1991;8:75–78.

28 Dastur DK, Dave UP. Effect of prolonged anticonvulsant medication in epileptic patients: serum lipids, vitamins B6, B12, and folic acid, proteins, and fine structure of liver. *Epilepsia* 1987;28:147–159.

29 Prakash PL, Singh G. Effects of folate supplementation on cleft palate induced by lamotrigine or cyclophosphamide: an experimental study in mice. *Neuroanatomy* 2007;6:12–16.

30 Sander JW, Patsalos PN. An assessment of serum and red blood cell folate concentrations in patients with epilepsy on lamotrigine therapy. *Epilepsy Res* 1992;13:89–92.

31 Phiel CJ, Zhang F, Huang EY, Guenther MG, Lazar MA, Klein PS. Histone deacetylase is a direct target of valproic acid, a potent anticonvulsant, mood stabilizer, and teratogen. *J Biol Chem* 2001;276:36734–36741.

32 Gottlicher M, Minucci S, Zhu P *et al*. Valproic acid defines a novel class of HDAC inhibitors inducing differentiation of transformed cells. *EMBO J* 2001;20:6969–6978.

33 Menegola E, Di Renzo F, Broccia ML *et al*. Inhibition of histone deacetylase activity on specific embryonic tissues as a new mechanism for teratogenicity. *Birth Defects Res B Dev Reprod Toxicol* 2005;74:392–398.

34 Eyal S, Yagen B, Sobol E, Altschuler Y, Shmuel M, Bialer M. The activity of antiepileptic drugs as histone deacetylase inhibitors. *Epilepsia* 2004;45:737–744.

35 Meador KJ, Penovich P, Baker GA *et al*. Antiepileptic drug use in women of childbearing age. *Epilepsy Behav* 2009;15:339–343.

36 Morrow J, Russell A, Guthrie E *et al*. Malformation risks of antiepileptic drugs in pregnancy: a prospective study from the UK Epilepsy and Pregnancy Register. *J Neurol Neurosurg Psychiatry* 2006;77:193–198.

37 Anderson GD, Yau MK, Gidal BE *et al*. Bidirectional interaction of valproate and lamotrigine in healthy subjects. *Clin Pharmacol Ther* 1996;60:145–156.

CHAPTER 13

Major Congenital Malformations in Offspring of Women with Epilepsy

Dina Battino[1] and Torbjörn Tomson[2]

[1] Epilepsy Centre, Department of Neurophysiology and Experimental Epileptology, IRCCS (Istituto di Ricovero a Cura a Carattere Scientifico) Neurological Institute "Carlo Besta" Foundation, Milan, Italy

[2] Department of Clinical Neuroscience, Karolinska Institutet, Stockholm, Sweden

> **Case history:** *This concerns a 28-year-old recently married school teacher. She has no family history of epilepsy and was perfectly healthy until 4 years ago when she experienced her first focal seizure. She experiences an auditory aura, which she finds difficult to describe, and after a few seconds impaired consciousness, which according to witnesses is accompanied by mild oral automatisms. She sought medical advice after her third similar seizure in 6 months. An EEG showed interictal epileptiform discharges over the right temporal region whereas magnetic resonance imaging (MRI) was completely normal. She was diagnosed with focal epilepsy of unknown cause (cryptogenic). Her physician started her on treatment with carbamazepine at gradually increasing dosages. She had a couple of additional identical seizures before becoming seizure-free on a carbamazepine dose of 400 mg twice daily, and she has now been completely seizure-free for 3 years on the medication. None of the five seizures were generalized. She is now considering pregnancy and consults her physician regarding risks and whether her treatment should be revised before pregnancy. There is no family history of congenital malformations.*

Introduction and background

Although the vast majority of women with epilepsy give birth to perfectly healthy children there is an increased risk of adverse pregnancy outcomes. These may include pregnancy losses, intrauterine growth retardation, impaired postnatal cognitive development, and increased prevalence of major congenital malformations. The reasons for the increased risks are multifactorial and may include genetic factors, the maternal epilepsy and seizures during pregnancy, socioeconomic status, and exposure to

Epilepsy in Women, First Edition. Edited by Cynthia L. Harden, Sanjeev V. Thomas and Torbjörn Tomson.

antiepileptic drugs (AEDs). Treatment decisions need to be based on considerations of all these possibilities but also need to take into account maternal risks associated with uncontrolled seizures. This chapter focuses on the risk of major congenital malformations in offspring of women with epilepsy, with emphasis on the role of AEDs and possible differences between drugs in their potential to cause major malformations. The other important aspects are covered in Chapters 8 and 9.

Major congenital malformations can be defined as structural abnormalities with surgical, medical, functional, or cosmetic importance. The definition usually excludes chromosomal or genetic abnormalities. Increased risk of congenital malformations among children of women with epilepsy was noted as early as the 1960s, when Meadow [1] reported hare-lip, cleft palate, and other abnormalities among babies of mothers who received primidone, phenytoin, or phenobarbital. He postulated that anticonvulsants should be added to the previously known factors that may cause such malformations. Numerous subsequent studies have confirmed a greater risk of major congenital malformations among children of mothers treated for epilepsy during pregnancy [2]. A systematic review and meta-analysis including 59 studies concluded that the overall prevalence of congenital malformations in children born of women with epilepsy is approximately threefold that of healthy women [3]. To what extent the greater risk is due to the exposure to AEDs or to other factors related to the maternal epilepsy was debated intensely over the decades following Meadow's early observations. In addition to the documented teratogenic effects of AEDs in preclinical screening models, there are clinical data that strongly support a major role for the AEDs for the increased risk. In a pooled analysis of data from 26 studies of outcomes of pregnancies of women with epilepsy, the malformation rate was 6.1% in offspring that had been exposed to AEDs (N=4630) compared with 2.8% in children of untreated women with epilepsy (N=1292) and 2.2% in offspring of mothers without epilepsy (N=40221) [4].

Similar results were reported in an earlier formal meta-analysis of 10 studies. The risk for congenital malformations in the offspring of women with untreated epilepsy was not higher than among nonepileptic controls [odds ratio (OR) 1.92; 95% CI 0.92–4.00]. The offspring of women with epilepsy who received AEDs had higher incidences of malformation than controls (OR 3.26; 95% CI 2.15–4.93) [5]. Further evidence comes from an association between drug load and malformation rates. Pooling data from 74 studies, the malformation rate was found to be 6.8% among those exposed to AEDs in polytherapy compared with 4.0% after monotherapy [4]. The afore-mentioned systematic review also found the highest malformation rate, 16.8%, among those exposed to polytherapy [3]. In monotherapy, the risk appears to depend on the prescribed dose. Increasing malformation rates with higher doses at the time of conception have been reported for valproic acid, carbamazepine, phenobarbital, and lamotrigine [6].

Although overwhelming data demonstrate that AEDs have the potential to cause major congenital malformations, most women with active epilepsy need to continue the treatment during pregnancy. The important question is therefore if AED treatment can differ in teratogenic potential and if women could choose a treatment that is effective and yet with minimized risks to the fetus. The emphasis in this chapter is on data from more recent studies comparing the risks for major malformations with different treatment options.

Some methodological considerations

Studies aiming at comparing the risks of malformations between different treatments face many challenges. First, and for obvious ethical reasons, pregnancy outcomes can never be assessed in randomized controlled studies. We generally have to rely on observational studies comparing pregnancy outcomes in women with different treatments. However, the women are not randomly allocated to their type of AED, or its dosage. The treatment choice is based on various individual characteristics including the maternal epilepsy syndrome and seizure severity, comorbidity, concomitant medication, educational level and other socioeconomic circumstances, and possibly also the family history of birth defects. Some of these AED selection criteria could also be risk factors for malformations and thus confound an observed association between exposure to a particular treatment and occurrence of malformations. As an example, having a parent with a major congenital malformation was independently associated with a more than four times greater risk in a large observational study of malformation rates after exposure to different AEDs [6]. Hence, an observed association between a particular drug and high malformation prevalence is not evidence of a causal relationship. Observational studies should thus try to obtain information on and control for possible confounders in the analyses. Second, to avoid reporting bias, information on exposure to treatment, as well as other risk factors, should be obtained before pregnancy outcome is known. However, with the more widespread use of early prenatal diagnostic tests, it is becoming increasingly difficult to enroll purely prospective pregnancies into observational studies before any information on fetal health is known. Third, as birth defects are fortunately also uncommon events in offspring of women with epilepsy, large patient materials are necessary. Fourth, an observed rate of malformations needs a comparison in order for it to be interpreted in a meaningful way. Whether this comparison group is children of healthy women, of mothers with untreated epilepsy, or of women treated with another AED, the controls have to be assessed in the same way as the exposed. Malformation rates vary depending on the population, the time period, and not least on criteria and methods for assessment. Historical or external controls are therefore not particularly useful.

The early reports of adverse pregnancy outcomes have traditionally been based on spontaneous reporting to pharmaceutical companies or regulatory authorities, or on series of cases collected in retrospect when outcome is known. Such reports may provide important signals, but cannot be used for proper risk assessment because of the risk of reporting bias. Physicians are more likely to report adverse than normal outcomes, and the total number of exposed is unknown. Such signals need to be confirmed or refuted in epidemiological studies that aim to establish if a birth defect occurs at a higher rate than expected after exposure to a specific AED. These studies typically utilize either a case–control or a cohort design. Case–control studies are particularly useful when the event of interest is rare, such as a specific uncommon birth defect. Cases with this birth defect are compared with controls, children without the defect, with regard to exposure to AEDs. In many case–control studies, the information on exposure is obtained after the pregnancy outcome is known, for example through interviews of the mothers after birth. There is an inherent risk of recall bias and an overestimation of risks in such studies. Case–control studies can provide a measure of the association between exposure to a particular treatment and birth defects, but they do not provide information on the frequency of the malformations in children exposed to the particular treatment or to comparators.

Cohort studies, on the other hand, evaluate outcome of pregnancies with a certain exposure, typically pregnancies in women with epilepsy on treatment with AEDs. Information on exposure in prospective cohort studies is ideally obtained before outcome is known, hence avoiding recall bias. It is not until recently, with the establishment of epilepsy and pregnancy registers, that sufficiently large cohort studies have become available [7]. The North American AED Pregnancy Registry (NAAPR) enrolls pregnant women from the USA and Canada. The UK Epilepsy and Pregnancy Register includes pregnancies from the UK and Ireland. EURAP is an international registry enrolling pregnant women from more than 40 countries worldwide. The Australian Pregnancy Register and the Kerala Registry of Epilepsy and Pregnancy in India are part of the EURAP collaboration but also publish independently [7]. Malformation rates after exposure to a specific treatment can be compared with rates after exposure to another treatment from the same cohort. Some epilepsy registers include an internal control group of unexposed nonepilepsy pregnancies. It is more problematic for the registers that are organized by a pharmaceutical company, for example the GlaxoSmithKline International Lamotrigine Register [7] or the UCB Keppra Registry [8], that only include pregnancies with the company's own product – one specific AED – without comparators [7]. Since methodologies and criteria vary slightly, it is also difficult to compare malformation rates and other outcomes between different epilepsy and pregnancy registries. Some Nordic countries have population-based nationwide registries including prospectively obtained exposure data as well as information on pregnancy outcome. Although not primarily designed to study AEDs, such registries have been used to assess risks associated with AEDs [9–12]. They have the advantage of data on outcome in the general population for comparison and their results are generalizable as they represent the whole country [7]. A limitation is the lack of detailed information on, for example, epilepsy type, seizure control, family history of birth defects, and drug dosage and other factors that could contribute to the outcome.

Major congenital malformations and AED exposure

Major congenital malformations include a wide variety of abnormalities with highly variable consequences for function and quality of life. Congenital malformations are established during organogenesis, largely equivalent to the first trimester. Sensitive periods vary with the type of malformation. Neural tube defects are established already during the third to fourth gestational week. Sensitive periods for congenital heart defects are weeks 4–8, and for orofacial clefts weeks 6–10. Malformations among offspring of women with epilepsy are not unique but generally follow a pattern similar to what is seen in the general population, with cardiac defects being the most common followed by facial clefts, and hypospadias. However, the patterns of malformations may vary with the type of AED. Studies in the 1980s and 1990s had already found an increase in the risk of neural tube defects specifically associated with maternal use of valproic acid [13,14] and possibly also of carbamazepine [15]. Table 13.1 lists the prevalence of some specific malformations in association with monotherapy exposure to five frequently used AEDs: carbamazepine, lamotrigine, barbiturates, phenytoin, and valproic acid. Studies included in Table 13.1 [6,12,16–19] are prospective, large, and fairly recent cohort studies. There are significant methodological differences between the included studies that could affect the pattern of malformations. As an example, selective exclusion of pregnancies with abnormal results on prenatal tests as in the UK Register will result in an underestimation of teratogenic risks and in particular of those malformations for which such tests are sensitive [17].

Table 13.1 Risk of some specific major congenital malformations by different monotherapies.

	All monotherapies (number of exposed)					Cardiovascular (per cent with malformation)					Hypospadias (per cent with malformation)					Oral clefts (per cent with malformation)					Neural tube defects (per cent with malformation)				
	CBZ	LTG	BA	PHT	VPA	CBZ	LTG	BA	PHT	VPA	CBZ	LTG	BA	PHT	VPA	CBZ	LTG	BA	PHT	VPA	CBZ	LTG	BA	PHT	VPA
Artama et al. [25]	805			38	263	0.4				1.5										1.9					1.9
Cunnington et al. [16]		1699					0.1					0.1					0.1					0.2			
North American Registry [28,29]			77		149			5.2							0.7			1.3							2.0
Kaaja et al. [18]	363	11		124	61		9.1			1.6	0.3			1.6		0.6			0.8		0.8				3.3
Morrow et al. [17]	927	684		85	762	0.6	0.6		1.2	0.7	0.2	0.9			1.2	0.4	1.5		1.5	1.5	0.2	0.1			0.9
Samrén et al. [19]	280		91	141	184			0.4	1.4	1.1	0.4			0.7	0.5	1.1		2.2			1.1				3.8
Wide et al. [12]	703	90	10	103	268	1.0				2.6	0.4				2.6	0.1				1.5	0.1				0.7
EURAP Registry [6]	989	781	217	89	678	1.9	0.9	2.8	2.2	2.5	0.9	0.5	0.5	101.1	2.5	0.2	0.3	0.5		0.6	0.5		0.5		
Total	4067	3254	406	580	2365																				

CBZ, carbamazepine; LTG, lamotrigine; BA, barbiturates; PHT, phenytoin; VPA, valproate.

Another example is different time windows for the assessment of the offspring. EURAP is assessing the occurrence of major malformations detected up to 1 year after birth and will thus identify malformations that are not apparent early after birth. Hence it is likely that internal malformations such as cardiac abnormalities are detected at higher rates in EURAP compared with the NAAPR or UK registries that assess outcome up to 2 months after birth [7]. Nevertheless, there are similarities in the patterns between the studies: cardiac malformations are the most common among offspring exposed to all AEDs and the risk appears particularly high with exposure to barbiturates; for all other included birth defects, the risk appears to be highest with exposure to valproic acid; and the prevalence of neural tube defects is particularly high with valproic acid.

NAAPR reported a prevalence of oral clefts of 7.3 per 1000 infants exposed to lamotrigine monotherapy, a 10-fold increased rate compared with unexposed infants [20]. The prevalence of oral clefts among lamotrigine-exposed infants was lower, 2.5 per 1000, in five other registries [20]. A case–control study utilizing the population-based EUROCAT database, which includes pregnancy outcomes with malformations in 14 European countries, investigated if first-trimester exposure to lamotrigine was specifically associated with an increased risk of orofacial clefts relative to other malformations [21]. This study found no evidence of a specific increased risk of orofacial clefts versus other malformations due to lamotrigine, but it was not designed to assess whether there is a general increased risk of malformations with lamotrigine [21]. NAAPR has also recently reported a 10-fold increase in the rate of orofacial clefts among infants exposed to topiramate monotherapy compared with unexposed infants [22]. As with lamotrigine, this is based on very few cases, and the observations have not yet been confirmed in other studies.

Case–control studies based on EUROCAT data have also investigated the risks for specific malformations in relation to first-trimester monotherapy exposure to valproic acid and carbamazepine. Compared with no use of an AED, exposure to valproic acid was associated with increased risks for spina bifida (OR 12.7; 95% CI 7.7–20.7), atrial septal defect (OR 2.5; 95% CI 1.4–4.4), cleft palate (OR 5.2; 95% CI 2.8–9.9), hypospadias (OR 4.8; 95% CI 2.9–8.1), polydactyly (OR 2.2; 95% CI 1.0–4.5), and craniosynostosis (OR 6.8; 95% CI 1.8–18.8) [23]. The only specific malformation associated with exposure to carbamazepine monotherapy was spina bifida (OR 2.6; 95% CI 1.2–5.3) compared with no AED [24]. Although these data can inform about associations between a particular AED and specific malformations, they rarely provide the direct comparison of risks between different drugs. Such comparative data are generally derived from the pregnancy registries and are usually confined to comparisons of overall malformations rates, since sample sizes are insufficient for across-drug comparisons of risks for specific malformations.

Rates of major congenital malformations with different monotherapy exposures from seven different registries are summarized in Table 13.2. The cohort studies included in the table have in common that information on exposure (use of AEDs in pregnancy) was obtained before pregnancy outcome was known, each included at least 500 pregnancies with monotherapy exposure, and all were published during the last decade [6,12,16–18,20,22,25–32].

The largest cohorts come from the three major independent epilepsy pregnancy registries, NAAPR, UK and EURAP. Initially, NAAPR released information on risks associated with exposure to specific AEDs when malformation rates were found to differ significantly from the rate among their external control population (1.6%). The malformation rates reported in Table 13.2 thus come from different publications released at different stages of the NAAPR study and do not represent a direct internal comparison between drugs. Increased malformation rates in comparison with the general population have so far been identified with phenobarbital [relative risk (RR) 4.2; 95% CI 1.5–9.4] (21) with a malformation rate of 6.5% based on 77 monotherapy exposures; and valproic acid (RR 7.3; 95% CI 4.4–12.2) (22) with a malformation rate of 10.7% (149 exposed). Subsequently, and based on new criteria, NAAPR reported malformation rates of 2.0% ($N=1562$) with lamotrigine monotherapy [31], 3.0% ($N=1033$) with carbamazepine [31], and 2.9% ($N=416$) with phenytoin monotherapy (31). The UK register data are based on 3607 cases [17]. The malformation rate after exposure to valproic acid monotherapy was 6.2% (4.6–8.2%) ($N=762$) compared with 2.2% (1.4–3.4%) for carbamazepine ($N=927$). The malformation rate with lamotrigine monotherapy was 3.2% (2.1–4.9%) based on 647 pregnancies. Among 227 children of women with untreated epilepsy the malformation rate was 3.5% (1.8–6.8%), similar to the 3.7% (3.0–4.5%) among the monotherapy exposures in general ($N=2468$). The UK Register has subsequently published outcome data on smaller samples of women treated with levetiracetam [26] and topiramate [27] (Table 13.2). EURAP recently published outcomes in pregnancies exposed to monotherapy with the most frequently used drugs [6]. The rate of major congenital malformations at 12 months after birth was 5.5% (4.4–6.8%) with carbamazepine ($N=1402$), 2.9% (2.0–4.0%) with lamotrigine ($N=1280$), 9.7% (7.9–11.7%) with valproic acid ($N=1010$), and 7.4% (4.3–11.7%) with phenobarbital ($N=217$). The risk of malformations with all these four investigated drugs was dose-dependent, which is discussed in more detail later. The Australian Register of Antiepileptic Drugs in Pregnancy collaborates with EURAP and feeds some pregnancies into EURAP, but also publishes independently. In its most recent update, the prevalence of malformations associated with monotherapy

Table 13.2 Overall rates of major congenital malformations (malformed/exposed) for different monotherapies.

Study	Carbamazepine	Lamotrigine	Phenobarbital	Phenytoin	Valproate	Gabapentin	Topiramate	Levetiracetam	Oxcarbazepine
Kaaja et al. [18]	10/363		0/5	3/124	4/61				1/9
Swedish Medical Birth Registry [12]	28/703	4/90	1/7	7/103	26/268	0/18			0/4
Finnish Drug prescription [25]	22/805			1/38	28/263				1/99
UK Register [17,26,27]	20/900	21/647		3/82	44/715	1/31	3/70	0/39	
International Lamotrigine Pregnancy Registry [16]		35/1558							
North American Registry [20,22,28–32]	31/1033	31/1562	11/199	12/416	30/317	1/145	15/359	11/450	4/182
EURAP Registry [6]	79/1402	37/1280	16/217	6/103	98/1010	0/23	5/73	2/126	6/184
Total	190/5206	128/5137	28/428	32/866	230/2634	2/217	23/502	13/615	12/478

with lamotrigine was 5.2% (*N*=231), 6.3% with carbamazepine (*N*=301), 16.3% with valproic acid (*N*=215), 2.9% with phenytoin (*N*=35), 3.2% with topiramate (*N*=31), and 0% with levetiracetam (*N*=22) [33]. The malformation rate among 116 offspring of untreated women with epilepsy was 5.2%. To avoid duplication these Australian data are not included in Table 13.2.

Studies from population-based nationwide generic registries from the Nordic countries have been complementary sources of information. Swedish, Finnish, Norwegian, and Danish Medical Birth registries have all been utilized to assess rates of malformations with exposure to different AEDs [9–12]. These registries provide observations that are representative of pregnancies of the unselected population taking AEDs in the country but include less information on possible confounding factors, including the maternal epilepsy, than the registries dedicated exclusively to epilepsy and pregnancy [7]. The Swedish Medical Birth Registry reported outcomes of 1398 pregnancies with exposure to AEDs regardless of indications [12]. The OR for having major congenital malformations among children exposed to monotherapy compared with all children of the general population was 1.61 (95% CI 1.18–2.19). The rate of malformations was higher after exposure to monotherapy with valproic acid compared with carbamazepine (OR 2.59; 95% CI 1.43–4.68). A study based on the Finnish Medical Birth and Drug Prescription Registries identified 1411 births where the women with epilepsy were using AEDs and 939 births among women with untreated epilepsy [11]. Congenital malformations were more common among offspring of women on AEDs (4.6%) than among offspring of untreated patients (2.8%). The malformation rate was higher with valproic acid monotherapy compared with children of untreated mothers with epilepsy (OR 4.18; 95% CI 2.31–7.57). There was no increase found among children exposed to carbamazepine, oxcarbazepine or phenytoin monotherapy, although the number of pregnancies with the two latter medications was low (Table 13.2) [11]. A study based on the Medical Birth Registry of Norway identified 961 pregnancies of women on medical treatment for their epilepsy [10]. This study did not report malformation rates with specific monotherapies, but only those exposed to valproic acid or polytherapy had increased rates of major malformations compared with nonepilepsy deliveries. The malformation rates were the same for infants of mothers with epilepsy that had been exposed to AEDs (2.7%) compared with mothers with untreated epilepsy (2.6%) if pregnancies with use of valproic acid were excluded [10]. The Danish Medical Birth Registry and other national health registries were utilized for a study with focus on newer-generation AEDs [9]. In total, 1532 with exposure to newer-generation AEDs during the first trimester were identified among 837 795 live births [9]. Unfortunately, this study also failed to distinguish between polytherapy and monotherapy. The rate of major malformations was 3.2% among children exposed to lamotrigine ($N=1019$), oxcarbazepine ($N=393$), topiramate ($N=108$), gabapentin ($N=59$), or levetiracetam ($N=58$) compared with 2.4% among the unexposed.

Table 13.2 also includes data from GlaxoSmithKline's International Lamotrigine Registry [16]. UCB Keppra Registry has so far reported 10 cases of major malformations among 227 children (4.4%) exposed to levetiraceteam in monotherapy [8]. For obvious reasons these data are difficult to interpret in the absence of a comparator.

As evident from Table 13.2 malformation rates vary across studies, reflecting differences in study populations, criteria and methodology, and demonstrating that rates should not be compared between studies. There is a fairly consistent pattern within studies, with higher rates with valproic acid and lower rates with carbamazepine and lamotrigine (Table 13.2). It is also evident that the number of monotherapy exposures with newer-generation drugs other than lamotrigine is too low to draw firm conclusions. However, even within-study comparisons should be made with some caution considering the possible effects of confounding factors. In the original publication from the UK Register, the statistical significance for observed lower malformation rates for lamotrigine compared with valproic acid exposures was lost after adjustment for age at birth, parity, family history of birth defects, folic acid use, and sex of infant [17]. EURAP included 10 nondrug covariates in a multivariable analysis. Parental history of major malformations was associated with a fourfold increased risk [6], demonstrating the importance of including such risk factors in the overall analysis.

EURAP systematically explored dose dependency and found that in monotherapy the risk of major congenital malformations increases dose dependently with all four assessed AEDs: carbamazepine, lamotrigine, valproic acid, and phenobarbital [6]. The dose dependency remained when 10 covariates were included in the multivariable analysis. The lowest malformation rates (2.0%, 1.19–3.24%) were observed with less than 300 mg/day of lamotrigine at the time of conception and with less than 400 mg/day of carbamazepine (3.4%, 1.11–7.71%). Malformation rates at different dosages of the four drugs in the EURAP study are summarized in Table 13.3. Doses of valproic acid below 700 mg/day were associated with a malformation rate in a similar range as that of carbamazepine 400–1000 mg/day, phenobarbital less than 150 mg/day, and lamotrigine 300 mg/day or higher.

Several previous studies have reported that the risk of malformations increases with the prescribed dose of valproic acid. Suggested cut-offs for

Table 13.3 Malformation rates (95% CI) of four monotherapies at different dose levels at time of conception.

AED (number exposed)	Dose range (mg/day)	Malformation rate (95% CI)
Carbamazepine (N=1402)	<400	3.4% (1.11–7.71)
	≥400 <1000	5.3% (4.07–6.89)
	≥1000	8.7% (5.24–13.39)
Lamotrigine (N=1280)	<300	2.0% (1.19–3.24)
	≥300	4.5% (2.77–6.87)
Phenobarbital (N=217)	<150	5.1% (2.51–10.04)
	≥150	13.7% (5.70–26.26)
Valproic acid (N=1010)	<700	5.6% (3.60–8.17)
	≥700 <1500	10.4% (7.83–13.50)
	≥1500	24.2% (16.19–33.89)

Source: data from EURAP Registry [6].

greater risks have varied from 600 to 1500 mg/day, although the criteria have rarely been accounted for [17,19,25,34–36]. The UK Pregnancy Register found greater risks of malformations with lamotrigine doses above 200 mg/day [17], this dose dependency was not confirmed in the North American or the International Lamotrigine Registry [16,20] but with some modification of the cut-off recently by EURAP [6]. These data support the general strategy of aiming at the lowest effective dose of an AED for women planning pregnancy.

As discussed above, most previous studies have reported higher rates of malformations with AEDs in polytherapy as compared with monotherapy [4]. However, more recent data clearly indicate that the risks associated with polytherapy depend on the AEDs that constitute the combination, and more specifically on the degree of exposure to valproic acid [37]. The Finnish Register-based study found that polytherapy without valproic acid was not associated with a significantly increased risk of malformations in relation to offspring of women with untreated epilepsy (OR 1.48; 95% CI 0.28–5.02) [25]. The UK Register concluded that polytherapies containing valproic acid in any combination had a significantly higher risk of major malformations than polytherapy combinations without valproic acid (OR 2.49; 95% CI 1.31–4.70) [17]. In NAAPR, lamotrigine monotherapy was associated with a malformation rate of 1.9%. The malformation rate with polytherapy including lamotrigine and valproic acid was 9.1%, whereas lamotrigine plus any other AED was associated with a rate of 2.9%. The rate of malformations was 2.9% with carbamazepine monotherapy, 15.4% in polytherapy with carbamazepine plus valproic acid, and 2.5% for carbamazepine plus any other AED [32].

Conclusions

During the last decade our knowledge concerning the risks of major congenital malformations in association with exposure to AEDs has increased substantially, in particular in relation to the three most frequently used drugs, carbamazepine, lamotrigine, and valproic acid. A major conclusion is that overall the increase in the risk with use of AEDs such as carbamazepine and lamotrigine in monotherapy is not as great as previously thought. On the other hand, valproic acid appears to be consistently associated with a greater risk than other AEDs whether used in monotherapy or as part of polytherapy. Although the pattern of malformations may be similar to that found in the general population, there are also examples of specific associations such as between exposure to valproic acid and neural tube defects. Importantly, these malformations are established in early pregnancy, often before the woman is aware of her pregnant state.

The risk of teratogenic effects appears to be dose-dependent. This has been most clearly demonstrated for valproic acid, where the risk increases at doses from 700 mg/day and above. These observations highlight the importance of trying out the lowest effective dose before conception.

Knowledge of the teratogenic potential of newer-generation AEDs other than lamotrigine is scarce. Although there are no signals of alarmingly high risks for major malformations with gabapentin, oxcarbazepine, levetiracetam, and topiramate, the data are insufficient for firm conclusions and for comparisons with other AEDs.

Review of the case: How should the available data affect the management of our case? This patient fortunately seeks advice in time, before pregnancy. Given that major congenital malformations are established in early pregnancy, treatment revision needs to be completed before pregnancy in order to possibly affect the risk. Also, the consequences of a seizure relapse that might be triggered by a treatment revision during pregnancy might adversely affect the fetus. Hence, treatment should be reviewed well in advance and any treatment revision completed and evaluated before conception. This might need up to a year including a slow gradual tapering of the drug. Our 28-year-old woman has been seizure-free for 3 years on monotherapy with carbamazepine 800 mg/day, a treatment associated with a modestly increased risk for birth defects. She has no demonstrable underlying pathology on MRI, and she entered remission rather quickly and on the first AED tried. Hence, the chance that she would remain seizure-free after withdrawal of carbamazepine is reasonably high. She is willing to take the risk of relapse and also to abstain from driving during the treatment revision. Carbamazepine is slowly reduced by 200 mg per month. She has a relapse with her habitual focal seizures 2 weeks after she reached a dose of 400 mg/day. The dose is therefore increased to 600 mg/day and she has remained seizure-free on that for 6 months when she becomes pregnant. The lowest effective dose of carbamazepine has thus been tried out in time before pregnancy.

> ○ **Key summary points**
> - The vast majority of women with epilepsy give birth to children without major congenital malformations.
> - There is a significant but modestly increased (1.5–2 fold) risk of major congenital malformations among offspring of women under AED treatment during pregnancy.
> - AED treatment is the major cause of the increased risk, but other factors (e.g., family history of birth defects) contribute.
> - The risk for major malformations is consistently higher with exposure to valproic acid compared with carbamazepine or lamotrigine.
> - Data on other newer-generation AEDs are still insufficient.
> - The risk of major malformations with the most frequently used AEDs appears to be dose-dependent.
> - Major malformations are established in early pregnancy and treatment revisions need to be considered, completed and evaluated before pregnancy to have a chance to be effective and safe.

References

1 Meadow SR. Anticonvulsant drugs and congenital abnormalities. *Lancet* 1968;ii:1296.
2 Harden CL, Meador KJ, Pennell PB *et al.* Practice Parameter update: management issues for women with epilepsy. Focus on pregnancy (an evidence-based review): teratogenesis and perinatal outcomes. Report of the Quality Standards Subcommittee and Therapeutics and Technology Subcommittee of the American Academy of Neurology and American Epilepsy Society. *Neurology* 2009;73:133–141.
3 Meador K, Reynolds MW, Crean S, Fahrbach K, Probst C. Pregnancy outcomes in women with epilepsy: a systematic review and meta-analysis of published pregnancy registries and cohorts. *Epilepsy Res* 2008;81:1–13.
4 Tomson T, Battino D. The management of epilepsy in pregnancy. In: Shorvon S, Pedley TA (eds) *The Blue Books of Neurology, The Epilepsies 3*. Philadelphia: Saunders Elsevier, 2009:241–264.
5 Fried S, Kozer E, Nulman I, Einarson TR, Koren G. Malformation rates in children of women with untreated epilepsy: a meta-analysis. *Drug Saf* 2004;27:197–202.
6 Tomson T, Battino D, Bonizzoni E *et al.* Dose-dependent risk of malformations with antiepileptic drugs: an analysis of data from the EURAP epilepsy and pregnancy registry. *Lancet Neurol* 2011;10:609–617.
7 Tomson T, Battino D, Craig J *et al.* Pregnancy registries: differences, similarities, and possible harmonization. *Epilepsia* 2010;51:909–915.
8 Montouris A, Harden C, Alekar S, Leppik I. UCB Antiepileptic Drug Pregnancy Registry Keppra® data [abstract]. 2010.
9 Molgaard-Nielsen D, Hviid A. Newer-generation antiepileptic drugs and the risk of major birth defects. *JAMA* 2011;305:1996–2002.
10 Veiby G, Daltveit AK, Engelsen BA, Gilhus NE. Pregnancy, delivery, and outcome for the child in maternal epilepsy. *Epilepsia* 2009;50:2130–2139.
11 Artama M, Ritvanen A, Gissler M, Isojarvi J, Auvinen A. Congenital structural anomalies in offspring of women with epilepsy: a population-based cohort study in Finland. *Int J Epidemiol* 2006;35:280–287.

12 Wide K, Winbladh B, Kallen B. Major malformations in infants exposed to antiepileptic drugs in utero, with emphasis on carbamazepine and valproic acid: a nationwide, population-based register study. *Acta Paediatr* 2004;93:174–176.

13 Lindhout D, Meinardi H. Spina bifida and in-utero exposure to valproate. *Lancet* 1984;ii:396.

14 Robert E, Guibaud P. Maternal valproic acid and congenital neural tube defects [Letter]. *Lancet* 1982;ii:937.

15 Kallen AJ. Maternal carbamazepine and infant spina bifida. *Reprod Toxicol* 1994;8:203–205.

16 Cunnington MC, Weil JG, Messenheimer JA, Ferber S, Yerby M, Tennis P. Final results from 18 years of the International Lamotrigine Pregnancy Registry. *Neurology* 2011;76:1817–1823.

17 Morrow J, Russell A, Guthrie E *et al*. Malformation risks of antiepileptic drugs in pregnancy: a prospective study from the UK Epilepsy and Pregnancy Register. *J Neurol Neurosurg Psychiatry* 2006;77:193–198.

18 Kaaja E, Kaaja R, Hiilesmaa V. Major malformations in offspring of women with epilepsy. *Neurology* 2003;60:575–579.

19 Samrén EB, van Duijn CM, Koch S *et al*. Maternal use of antiepileptic drugs and the risk of major congenital malformations: a joint European prospective study of human teratogenesis associated with maternal epilepsy. *Epilepsia* 1997;38:981–990.

20 Holmes LB, Baldwin EJ, Smith CR *et al*. Increased frequency of isolated cleft palate in infants exposed to lamotrigine during pregnancy. *Neurology* 2008;70:2152–2158.

21 Dolk H, Jentink J, Loane M, Morris J, de Jong-van den Berg LT. Does lamotrigine use in pregnancy increase orofacial cleft risk relative to other malformations? *Neurology* 2008;71:714–722.

22 Hernandez Diaz R, Mittendorf R, Holmes L. Comparative safety of topiramate during pregnancy [Abstract]. *Birth Defects Res A Clin Mol Teratol* 2010;88:408.

23 Jentink J, Loane MA, Dolk H *et al*. Valproic acid monotherapy in pregnancy and major congenital malformations. *N Engl J Med* 2010;362:2185–2193.

24 Jentink J, Dolk H, Loane MA *et al*. Intrauterine exposure to carbamazepine and specific congenital malformations: systematic review and case-control study. *Br Med J* 2010;341:c6581.

25 Artama M, Auvinen A, Raudaskoski T, Isojarvi I, Isojarvi J. Antiepileptic drug use of women with epilepsy and congenital malformations in offspring. *Neurology* 2005;64:1874–1878.

26 Hunt S, Craig J, Russell A *et al*. Levetiracetam in pregnancy: preliminary experience from the UK Epilepsy and Pregnancy Register. *Neurology* 2006;67:1876–1879.

27 Hunt S, Russell A, Smithson WH *et al*. Topiramate in pregnancy: preliminary experience from the UK Epilepsy and Pregnancy Register. *Neurology* 2008;71:272–276.

28 Holmes LB, Wyszynski DF, Lieberman E. The AED (antiepileptic drug) pregnancy registry: a 6-year experience. *Arch Neurol* 2004;61:673–678.

29 Wyszynski DF, Nambisan M, Surve T, Alsdorf RM, Smith CR, Holmes LB. Increased rate of major malformations in offspring exposed to valproate during pregnancy. *Neurology* 2005;64:961–965.

30 Hernandez-Diaz S, Smith CR, Wyszynski DF, Holmes LB. Risk of major malformations among infants exposed to carbamazepine during pregnancy. *Birth Defects Res A Clin Mol Teratol* 2007;79:357.

31 Hernandez-Diaz S, Smith CR, Shen A *et al*. Comparative safety of antiepileptic drugs during pregnancy. *Neurology* 2012;78:1692–1699.

32 Holmes LB, Mittendorf R, Shen A, Smith CR, Hernandez-Diaz S. Fetal effects of anticonvulsant polytherapies: different risks from different drug combinations. *Arch Neurol* 2011;68:1275–1281.

33 Vajda FJ, Graham J, Roten A, Lander CM, O'Brien TJ, Eadie M. Teratogenicity of the newer antiepileptic drugs: the Australian experience. *J Clin Neurosci* 2012;19:57–59.

34 Kaneko S, Battino D, Andermann E *et al*. Congenital malformations due to antiepileptic drugs. *Epilepsy Res* 1999;33:145–158.

35 Samrén EB, van Duijn CM, Christiaens GC, Hofman A, Lindhout D. Antiepileptic drug regimens and major congenital abnormalities in the offspring. *Ann Neurol* 1999;46:739–746.

36 Vajda FJ, Hitchcock A, Graham J, O'Brien T, Lander C, Eadie M. The Australian Register of Antiepileptic Drugs in Pregnancy: the first 1002 pregnancies. *Aust NZ J Obstet Gynaecol* 2007;47:468–474.

37 Vajda FJ, Hitchcock AA, Graham J, O'Brien TJ, Lander CM, Eadie MJ. The teratogenic risk of antiepileptic drug polytherapy. *Epilepsia* 2010;51:805–810.

CHAPTER 14

Fetal AED Syndromes

Usha Kini

Department of Clinical Genetics, The Churchill Hospital, Oxford, UK

Case history: *Mrs H. was diagnosed with epilepsy, following a car accident, when she was 13 years old. She was treated with valproate and lamotrigine to control her seizures. During her first pregnancy, she took 700 mg/day of valproate and 150 mg/day of lamotrigine throughout the pregnancy. She took normal-dose folic acid (0.4 mg/day) from 8 weeks of pregnancy when she found she was pregnant. Her daughter was born healthy and continued to develop normally.*

Prior to her second pregnancy, the dose of valproate was increased to 1200 mg/day to help control her seizures. She took 0.4 mg/day of folic acid when she was 5 weeks' pregnant and continued it throughout the pregnancy. A fetal cardiac scan at 18 weeks showed that the baby had a bicuspid aortic valve. An amniocentesis was carried out to rule out Down syndrome and other common trisomies. Her son, A.H., was born at term and weighed 2.353 kg. He was noted to be dysmorphic with a prominent metopic suture, thin arched eyebrows, broad nasal bridge, anteverted nose, infraorbital grooves, smooth long philtrum, and thin upper lip. He was also noted to have left preaxial polydactyly and hypospadias, both of which were surgically treated. The metopic synostosis was surgically treated when he was 2 years of age. He did not need further follow-up for his bicuspid aortic valve.

A.H. has global developmental delay. He started walking at the age of 3 years and receives physiotherapy. At the age of 3.5 years, he has 10–12 single words in his speech. His vision is normal but there are concerns about his hearing and he has been found to have serous otitis media in both his ears. There are no concerns about his behavior. Investigations that were reported to be normal included chromosomes, fragile X testing and array CGH (comparative genomic hybridization).

Mrs H. did not receive pre-pregnancy counseling for either pregnancy.

Background and important details

Fetal AED syndrome is a term used to describe a pattern of abnormalities occurring together, including facial dysmorphism, congenital malformations, developmental delay, learning difficulties, and behavioral problems, in a child with prenatal exposure to antiepileptic drugs (AEDs). Not all

---

Epilepsy in Women, First Edition. Edited by Cynthia L. Harden, Sanjeev V. Thomas and Torbjörn Tomson.

affected individuals show all the features. Exposure to specific AEDs such as valproate, phenytoin and carbamazepine may cause specific abnormalities and then the terms 'fetal valproate syndrome' (FVS), 'fetal phenytoin syndrome' or 'fetal carbamazepine syndrome' may be used. Some women may be on more than one AED during the pregnancy, when use of the term 'fetal AED syndrome' would be more appropriate.

FVS is the best-described syndrome of all the fetal AED syndromes, as valproate is the most teratogenic and is frequently used in the treatment of epilepsy. Valproate is also used in the treatment of psychiatric illnesses such as bipolar disorders. The teratogenic effects of valproate are likely to occur when the dose during pregnancy is 1000 mg/day and above [1,2].

The first case of teratogenicity with valproate was reported in 1980. Di Liberti *et al.* [3] coined the term 'fetal valproate syndrome' in 1984 following several other reports of teratogenicity with this drug. The facial dysmorphism of FVS includes a prominent metopic ridge, thin arched eyebrows with medial deficiency, epicanthic folds, infraorbital grooves, broad nasal bridge, short anteverted nose, smooth long philtrum, and a thin upper lip [4]. These features are better appreciated in infancy and become less obvious with age. It is often the facial gestalt rather than the individual features that provide a clue to the diagnosis [5].

Several congenital malformations have been reported in FVS and are discussed in more detail in Chapter 13. The most specific malformations include neural tube defects, trigonocephaly, radial ray defects, pulmonary abnormalities, and colobomata of the iris and retinae [6], although some of these are rare.

Developmental delay, especially affecting speech, is common in FVS. The speech and language problems continue later in life and are reflected as lower verbal IQ compared with performance IQ [7]. Children with FVS may have additional educational needs and require extra help at school [8]. Behavioral problems such as autistic spectrum disorder and poor attention and hyperactivity have been reported with increased frequency [9].

Fetal carbamazepine syndrome is caused by prenatal exposure to carbamazepine and has not been found to be dose-dependent. However, the features of fetal carbamazepine syndrome are subtle. The facial gestalt has been described as a 'doll-like facies' and consists of features such as full cheeks, small chin, and everted lower lip [5]. Congenital malformations may occur (described in Chapter 13) but are not specific to carbamazepine exposure. The frequency of neural tube defects is increased about fivefold compared with the general population. Microcephaly (head circumference below the 3rd centile) has been noted. Developmental delay may be seen but tends to be mild and may affect any area of development. Several studies have shown that the IQ of children with *in utero* exposure to carbamazepine is within the normal range [10].

Fetal phenytoin syndrome was first described by Loughnan *et al.* in 1973 [11] and expanded upon by Hanson and Smith in 1976 [12]. The features noted were hypertelorism, a broad flat nasal bridge, an upturned nasal tip, distal digital hypoplasia, and hirsutism.

Monotherapy with the newer AEDs such as lamotrigine, levetiracetam and topiramate given has been thought to have teratogenic effects. However, the severity and frequency of the teratogenic effects appear to be less than those caused by exposure to valproate. The evidence is new and limited, but some studies have shown that while these drugs may cause a slightly increased risk of congenital abnormalities [13], they may not affect the facial appearance or the intellect and behavior [14,15]. Further studies are needed to confirm this.

Treatment with polytherapy is reported to have a more adverse outcome on the fetus [16]. It is difficult to deduce which features may be related to a particular AED exposure as there is much overlap between the effects of different AEDs. The outcome appears to be worse when valproate forms part of the polytherapy [17]. There has been increasing recognition that the facial gestalt may be a helpful predictor of learning difficulties in those with obvious dysmorphism [5].

Implications for management

Fetal AED syndrome is a diagnosis of exclusion as there are no objective tests that may confirm the diagnosis. Several chromosome abnormalities, genetic disorders like fragile X syndrome, and other fetal insults such as alcohol and toluene exposure may result in clinical features similar to those seen in fetal AED syndromes. Karyotyping, testing for fragile X syndrome, and array CGH (comparative genomic hybridization for detailed chromosome analysis) should be offered wherever possible before making the diagnosis.

When considering the management of fetal AED syndromes, two important aspects need to be kept in mind: (i) the active treatment and screening of the problems known to be associated with fetal AED syndrome and (ii) the prevention of recurrence of fetal AED syndrome in a future pregnancy.

Active treatment and screening

Surgical intervention may be needed for specific congenital malformations such as heart defects, metopic synostosis (trigonocephaly), hypospadias, limb defects, and so on. Echocardiogram, ultrasound scan of the kidneys, and ophthalmological examination should be offered early to those suspected of having fetal AED syndrome. Childhood medical problems such as refractive errors of vision and recurrent serous otitis media are common and hence regular monitoring of vision and audiological assessments should be offered. Physiotherapy, speech and language therapy, and occupational therapy should be made available to those with developmental delay in order to help them achieve their full potential. Extra help at school should be provided early to those displaying developmental delay. Behavioral therapy and medication may help in those with behavioral problems.

There is a slightly increased risk of epilepsy (about 4%) in the offspring of a parent with epilepsy [18]. This is unrelated to the AED exposure but should be monitored for and treated early.

Prevention of recurrence

The risk of recurrence of fetal AED syndrome is low if the maternal medication is changed. All women with epilepsy should receive pre-pregnancy counseling. It is advisable to be on monotherapy rather than polytherapy and the dose of the AED should be reduced to the minimal level required to control the seizures. Use of valproate should be avoided if possible. In cases where this cannot be achieved every effort should be made to reduce the dose below 1000 mg/day. All changes to the drugs and their dose should always be made in liaison with the doctor. The occurrence of seizures during pregnancy can be detrimental to the health of the fetus and the mother (e.g., sudden unexpected death in epilepsy or SUDEP).

For women on AEDs, high-dose folic acid (4 mg/day), which is available by prescription, is recommended starting 6 weeks prior to becoming pregnant and throughout the first trimester at least [19], with the aim of reducing the risk of congenital malformations. As the fetal brain continues to grow throughout pregnancy, it may be advisable to take folic acid until delivery.

In pregnant women, antenatal scans are able to pick up structural abnormalities at about 18–20 weeks. Subtle abnormalities such as a cleft palate may be missed on scanning. Gross abnormalities such as anencephaly may be identified on earlier scans (e.g., a dating scan). Fetal cardiac scans should also be offered. Serum alpha-fetoprotein may be tested at 15 weeks to look for open neural tube defects.

Review of the case: Mrs H. is a woman with epilepsy who took AEDs during both her pregnancies for control of her epilepsy. She was on polytherapy during both pregnancies but the dose of valproate was increased above 1000 mg/day prior to the second pregnancy. Because of the lack of pre-pregnancy counseling, high-dose folic acid had not been recommended. Also, no attempt had been made to reduce the number of antiepileptic medications she was using, prior to the pregnancy.

Mrs H. was at higher risk of having a child with fetal AED syndrome due to the use of polytherapy, of which valproate was a part. The dose of valproate during the second pregnancy was more than 1000 mg/day, increasing her risk further.

A.H. showed the facial features associated with FVS. He also had congenital abnormalities that are specifically associated with valproate exposure, namely metopic synostosis and radial ray defect (preaxial polydactyly). He also has global developmental delay needing additional support in the form of physiotherapy and speech therapy.

Following the diagnosis in A.H., Mrs H. has been referred to a neurologist for review of the AEDs and the dose of valproate that she is using currently. Any change in her medication will have to be carried out prior to another pregnancy. She has also been advised to take high-dose folic acid from the time she starts to plan her pregnancy until the delivery. Mrs H. is worried that if her seizures return while her AEDs are being altered, she may lose her driving license. This will impact on her daily activities. This will have to be taken into account when changing her AED dose.

Key summary points

- Fetal AED syndrome refers to the pattern of teratogenic effects caused by prenatal exposure to AEDs.

- The teratogenic effects include major structural malformations, minor anomalies including dysmorphic facial features, childhood medical problems, developmental delay, additional educational needs, and behavioral problems.

- Valproate is the most teratogenic AED known and has a dose-dependent effect (>1000 mg/day).

- Polytherapy is more teratogenic than monotherapy, particularly when valproate is part of the polytherapy.

- Pre-pregnancy counseling and reassessment of the AED medication is very important in women with epilepsy to reduce the risk of fetal AED syndrome.

- High-dose folic acid is recommended during the pregnancy in women with epilepsy and should be started at least 6 weeks prior to pregnancy and continued throughout the pregnancy.

References

1 Battino D, Binelli S, Caccamo ML *et al*. Malformations in offspring of 305 epileptic women: a prospective study. *Acta Neurol Scand* 1992;85:204–207.
2 Mawer G, Clayton-Smith J, Coyle H, Kini U. Outcome of pregnancy in women attending an outpatient epilepsy clinic: adverse features associated with higher doses of sodium valproate. *Seizure* 2002;11:512–518.
3 DiLiberti JH, Farndon PA, Dennis NR, Curry CJ. The fetal valproate syndrome. *Am J Med Genet* 1984;19:473–481.
4 Clayton-Smith J, Donnai D. Fetal valproate syndrome. *J Med Genet* 1995;32:724–727.
5 Kini U, Adab N, Vinten J, Fryer A, Clayton-Smith J; Liverpool Manchester Neurodevelopmental Study Group. Dysmorphic features: an important clue to the diagnosis and severity of fetal anticonvulsant syndromes. *Arch Dis Child* 2006;91:F90–F95.
6 Kini U. Fetal valproate syndrome: a review. *Paediatr Perinat Drug Ther* 2006;7:123–130.

7 Adab N, Kini U, Vinten J *et al.* The longer term outcome of children born to mothers with epilepsy. *J Neurol Neurosurg Psychiatry* 2004;75:1575–1583.

8 Adab N, Jacoby A, Smith D, Chadwick D. Additional educational needs in children born to mothers with epilepsy. *J Neurol Neurosurg Psychiatry* 2001;70:15–21.

9 Vinten J, Adab N, Kini U, Gorry J, Gregg J, Baker GA; Liverpool Manchester Neurodevelopmental Study Group. Neuropsychological effects of exposure to anticonvulsant medication in utero. *Neurology* 2005;64:949–954.

10 Gaily E, Kantola-Sorsa E, Hiilesmaa V *et al.* Normal intelligence in children with prenatal exposure to carbamazepine. *Neurology* 2004;62:28–32.

11 Loughnan PM, Gold H, Vance JC. Phenytoin teratogenicity in man. *Lancet* 1973; i:70–72.

12 Hanson JW, Smith DW. Fetal hydantoin syndrome. *Lancet* 1976;i:692.

13 Vajda FJ, Graham J, Roten A, Lander CM, O'Brien TJ, Eadie M. Teratogenicity of the newer antiepileptic drugs: the Australian experience. *J Clin Neurosci* 2012;19:57–59.

14 Meador KJ, Baker GA, Browning N *et al.* Cognitive function at 3 years of age after fetal exposure to antiepileptic drugs. *N Engl J Med* 2009;360:1597–1605.

15 Shallcross R, Bromley RL, Irwin B, Bonnett LJ, Morrow J, Baker GA; Liverpool Manchester Neurodevelopment Group; UK Epilepsy and Pregnancy Register. Child development following in utero exposure: levetiracetam vs sodium valproate. *Neurology* 2011;76:383–389.

16 Kaneko S, Battino D, Andermann E *et al.* Congenital malformations due to antiepileptic drugs. *Epilepsy Res* 1999;33:145–158.

17 Holmes LB, Mittendorf R, Shen A, Smith CR, Hernandez-Diaz S. Fetal effects of anticonvulsant polytherapies: different risks from different drug combinations. *Arch Neurol* 2011;68:1275–1281.

18 Harper P. Central nervous system disorders. In: *Practical Genetic Counselling*, 6th edn. London: Hodder Arnold, 2004: 183–185.

19 Crawford P, Appleton R, Betts T, Duncan J, Guthrie E, Morrow J. Best practice guidelines for the management of women with epilepsy. The Women with Epilepsy Guidelines Development Group. *Seizure* 1999;8:201–217.

CHAPTER 15

Postnatal Cognitive Development

Evan R. Gedzelman and Kimford J. Meador

Department of Neurology, Emory University School of Medicine, Atlanta, Georgia, USA

Case history: *A 25-year-old woman is referred for management. She is pregnant at an estimated 8 weeks gestation. At age 15 years she experienced a generalized tonic–clonic seizure (GTCS) without warning. An EEG was reported to show a single discharge at the right frontal lobe, and magnetic resonance imaging (MRI) was reported as normal. She was treated with phenytoin but developed a rash, then treated with carbamazepine and later topiramate, but suffered a GTCS with each. She was then switched to valproate and remained seizure-free. She has never had separate myoclonic jerks, and family history is negative for epilepsy. Several months ago, she married and moved to a local community. She established care with a new neurologist. A repeat EEG was normal. Since she was planning a pregnancy, the new neurologist slowly titrated her onto lamotrigine to a target dose of 100 mg b.i.d. and then tapered off the valproate. Three days after stopping the valproate a convulsion occurred, and valproate was restarted at her previous dose. Shortly thereafter she became pregnant for the first time. Her present medications are generic lamotrigine 100 mg b.i.d. and valproate (Divalproex sodium) 250 mg b.i.d. Anticonvulsant blood levels are lamotrigine 4.0 µg/dL and valproate 42 µg/dL. Her medical history is otherwise unremarkable. Her neurological exam is normal. Another EEG is normal.*

Background

In children of women with epilepsy, a multitude of factors may contribute to observed neurodevelopmental deficits. These include antiepileptic drugs (AEDs), seizures during pregnancy, seizure type, heredity, maternal age/parity, and socioeconomic status [1,2]. AEDs play an important role in this regard as suggested by data from animals and humans, although many issues remain unresolved [3].

Epilepsy in Women, First Edition. Edited by Cynthia L. Harden, Sanjeev V. Thomas and Torbjörn Tomson.

© 2013 John Wiley & Sons, Ltd. Published 2013 by John Wiley & Sons, Ltd.

Cognitive effects of maternal epilepsy in absence of AEDs during pregnancy

No IQ difference was found between children of untreated women with epilepsy and healthy controls based on both a prospective blinded and observational study [4] and a blinded retrospective study [5].

Cognitive effects of maternal seizures during pregnancy

Two prospective population-based studies found no IQ impairment in children exposed *in utero* to self-limiting (i.e., no status epilepticus) GTCS [4,6]. However, in children exposed to more than four GTCS, verbal IQ was significantly reduced based on one retrospective study [7]. Case reports have documented that prolonged seizures and status epilepticus are a serious threat to both mother and fetus [8].

Cognitive effects of fetal AED exposure

The impact of *in utero* exposure to AEDs on cognitive and behavioral development has recently emerged as an area of concern. Maternal use of some AEDs during pregnancy may negatively impact cognition in infants of women with epilepsy. This is suggested by research efforts thus far [9]. Even though much progress has been made recently in developing pregnancy registries, evaluation and comparison of reports on AED teratogenicity, cognitive outcomes, and behavioral outcomes are difficult. Outcome data are incomplete. Registries are observational investigations, deal with different cultures and populations, have variable methodology, have different definitions, have different standardized tests (e.g., different cognitive tests), and have variable follow-up times. The registries also vary in their data collection timing (e.g., major congenital malformations at birth vs. at 1 year old). A dearth of information about mothers in addition to a lack of follow-up restricts usefulness of registry data. Additionally, individual registries have weaknesses ranging from missing data on key variables to low numbers for specific AEDs [10]. Given these limitations, in order to be confident of results, the signals for specific AEDs need to be reproduced in more than one registry.

Other factors

One study showed that low maternal IQ, maternal education, and antenatal AED exposure were all associated with significant impairment of intellectual and language functions at 6 years old. This study was drawn from a prospective cohort in the Kerala Registry of Epilepsy and Pregnancy with 201 children of parents without epilepsy used as matched controls (for age and socioeconomic status). It utilized an Indian adaptation of the Wechsler Intelligence Scale for children and a locally developed proficiency test for regional language [11].

Pregnancy outcomes with regard to neurodevelopment

Effects of fetal AED exposure on neurodevelopment

It has become evident based on animal studies that fetal exposure to AEDs at doses lower than the threshold required to produce congenital malformations can produce cognitive and behavioral abnormalities [12]. The notion that AED exposure during fetal development can produce behavioral defects that can occur at dosages lower than those required to produce somatic malformations is supported by additional studies [13,14]. Exposure to AEDs in the gestational or neonatal period can alter brain chemistry, reduce brain weight, delay neurodevelopment, cause hyperactivity, and impair behavior, motor coordination and memory [15].

Possible mechanisms of behavioral teratogenesis

A teratogen has its most profound impact on a susceptible genotype, and this effect may involve the interaction of multiple-liability genes [16]. For example, discordant outcomes have been witnessed in dizygotic twin fetuses exposed to phenytoin [17]. The mechanisms involved in both behavioral and anatomical defects may be dissimilar since anatomical risks are related to first-trimester exposure, but behavioral deficits may be related primarily to third-trimester exposure. Proposed possible mechanisms underlying functional/behavioral teratogenicity of AEDs include folate, reactive intermediates (e.g., epoxides or free radicals), ischemia, apoptosis-related mechanisms, neuronal suppression, and alterations to neurotransmitter systems [3].

Reactive intermediates

Toxic intermediary metabolites and not necessarily the parent compound may mediate the fetotoxicity of some AEDs [18]. These medications may be bioactivated to form free-radical reactive intermediates by embryonic prostaglandin H synthetase or lipoxygenases [19–21]. Once formed, these free radical reactive oxygen species may bind to protein, lipids, or even DNA, resulting in teratogenesis [3].

Ischemia/hypoxia

Ischemia-induced embryopathy in animals resembles phenytoin-induced defects in humans. In addition, hyperoxic chamber treatment is known to reduce malformations caused by phenytoin [22]. However, the similarity to AED-induced defects may alternatively be caused by free radical-induced ischemia [3].

Folate

DNA and RNA synthesis requires folate, and during pregnancy this demand is increased. Of the major enzyme inducer AEDs, phenobarbital, phenytoin and primidone, but not carbamazepine, deplete folate [23–26]. Valproate also affects folate-dependent one-carbon metabolism [27]. In women with epilepsy who have abnormal pregnancy outcomes, blood folate concentrations were found to be significantly lower [28]. In addition, infants of women with epilepsy who received no folate supplementation had a 15% rate of malformation according to Biale and Lewenthal [29]. No congenital abnormalities were identified in 33 folate-supplemented children in the study [3].

Neuronal suppression

AEDs suppress neuronal irritability and as a result impair neuronal excitation. *In utero* reduction of neuronal excitation could modify synaptic growth and connectivity in early stages of neurodevelopment. This in turn could result in long-term deficits in cognition and behavior [3].

Apoptosis-related mechanisms

Ethanol can produce widespread neuronal apoptosis that leads to neurobehavioral deficits in the developing brain [30]. Ethanol can also produce neuronal dysfunction in the remaining neurons [31]. These results led to adoption of the apoptotic model in studies with AEDs. In the neonatal rat brain, AEDs that have been observed to produce widespread neuronal apoptosis include valproate, vigabatrin, phenytoin, phenobarbital, diazepam, and clonazepam [32–36]. The effect occurs at therapeutically relevant blood levels, can occur with just a single dose exposure, and is dose-dependent. The effect is also synergistic because two AEDs, given at below threshold dosages, can still trigger the full apoptotic response. Several AEDs can enhance apoptosis induced by another one, even though the particular AED does not produce apoptosis itself in monotherapy [37]. These include lamotrigine, carbamazepine, and topiramate [38–40]. These findings suggest that polytherapy could increase the risk. Levetiracetam is the only AED of those tested so far that neither produces apoptosis in monotherapy nor enhances apoptosis of other AEDs [39]. However, most AEDs have not been tested. The results from these animal experiments raise concern that commonly used AEDs could lead to similar adverse effects in children of women with epilepsy exposed *in utero*. However, clinical studies are required to confirm if similar effects occur in the human brain.

Alterations to neurotransmitter systems

Both neuronal proliferation and migration can be affected by AED alterations to neurotransmitter systems. Glutamate action is inhibited by multiple AEDs including felbamate and topiramate. Agonists of γ-aminobutyric acid (GABA) include phenobarbital, benzodiazepines, and valproate. The neurotransmitter medium in the developing brain regulates neuronal differentiation and migration. Blockade of N-methyl-D-aspartate (NMDA) receptors or enhanced GABA inhibition impairs neurogenesis and cell migration based on animal studies [35,41]. This can result in decreased brain volume and cortical dysplasias. Enhanced GABA activity [42] or drug-induced inhibition of NMDA receptor activity [43] can disrupt the process of synaptogenesis. Impaired cognition in children exposed *in utero* to AEDs may be due to these neurotransmitter changes and subsequent cellular changes [9].

Neurodevelopmental effects of individual AEDs

Carbamazepine

No effect of fetal carbamazepine exposure on IQ was reported in a prospective, evaluator-blinded, observational study with matched controls [44]. No adverse effects of fetal carbamazepine exposure were seen in a population-based, longitudinal, follow-up study of preschool children [45]. A retrospective blinded study controlling for maternal IQ in 52 children of women with epilepsy exposed to carbamazepine versus 80 unexposed children found no IQ difference [46]. Similarly, no IQ difference was seen in 86 children of women with epilepsy exposed to carbamazepine monotherapy versus 45 children of women with epilepsy on no AED or 141 healthy control children in a prospective, population-based, blinded, observational study controlling for maternal education [4]. When these data were pooled with data from another prospective population-based study, only one of 84 children exposed to polytherapy exhibited mental retardation [4,6]. Again, no IQ difference was seen in children of women with epilepsy exposed to carbamazepine versus no AED in another population-based, evaluator-blinded study [47]. Eighty children exposed to carbamazepine monotherapy showed no difference in frequency of autism spectrum from the general population according to a retrospective population-based study [48]. In a prospective observational multicenter study, children at age 3 who had been previously exposed to carbamazepine *in utero* did not differ from the lamotrigine- or phenytoin-exposed groups, although they had better IQ outcomes than the valproate group [49]. Based on the same study, a follow-up investigation showed fetal exposure to carbamazepine was associated with a dose-related reduction in language abilities at age 3 and again at age 4.5 [12,50].

Lamotrigine

In a prospective observational study, children at age 3 exposed *in utero* to lamotrigine did not differ from those exposed to carbamazepine or phenytoin, but had better IQ outcomes than those exposed to valproate at age 3 [49]. Dose-related effects of fetal AED exposure on verbal and non-verbal cognitive measures were assessed in exposed 3-year-old children in a follow-up investigation [12]. This study set out to ascertain if differential long-term neurodevelopmental effects occur across four commonly utilized AEDs (carbamazepine, lamotrigine, phenytoin, and valproate). The Differential Ability Scales, Preschool Language Scale, Peabody Picture Vocabulary Test and Developmental Test of Visual–Motor Integration were used to calculate cognitive outcomes in 216 children. Children exposed *in utero* to each drug had lower verbal abilities than nonverbal for all four AEDs, but no dose effects were seen for lamotrigine and phenytoin [12].

Levetiracetam

A recent study reported that children exposed to levetiracetam obtained higher developmental scores at under 24 months of age when compared with children exposed to valproate. This study compared levetiracetam to valproate and to a control group (levetiracetam, $N=51$; valproate, $N=44$; $P<0.001$). The levetiracetam group did not differ from the controls ($N=97$; $P=0.62$) [51]. The limitations of the study included (i) completer rates of only 58% for levetiracetam and 37% for valproate, (ii) young age at assessment, and (iii) retrospective collection of some data. Replication of these findings is needed. Caution should be exercised when utilizing this source for clinical application given these limitations and given that this is the only study on the neurodevelopmental effects of levetiracetam.

Phenobarbital

No difference in IQ was seen in 35 children of women with epilepsy exposed *in utero* to phenobarbital monotherapy versus 4705 children of mothers without epilepsy based on a study published in 1976 [52]. In contrast to this report, two studies of separate cohorts of 114 adult men exposed *in utero* to phenobarbital (of mothers without epilepsy) found approximately 0.5 standard deviations lower verbal IQ scores in the exposed group [53]. Young children exposed to phenobarbital have been shown to have statistically different IQ compared with control groups. Though not an investigation of fetal exposure, one study of phenobarbital use in young children with febrile seizures offers insights into the effects of phenobarbital on the immature brain. A total of 217 children with febrile seizures were randomized to either a phenobarbital or placebo group, and tested 2 years later; those in the phenobarbital group demonstrated lower IQ [54]. In order to reduce the risk of poor cognitive outcomes, avoidance of phenobarbital in women with epilepsy during pregnancy, if possible, may be considered [55].

Phenytoin

No effect of fetal phenytoin exposure on IQ was seen in two prospective, blinded, population-based studies that controlled for maternal education level or socioeconomic class [6,52]. Another study of the same design, but drawn from a different patient pool, demonstrated lower IQ at age 7 years in children of women with epilepsy exposed to phenytoin versus healthy control children of mothers without epilepsy [56]. Slightly lower scores for locomotor development were reported in preschool children in phenytoin-exposed children versus fetal carbamazepine-exposed children and unexposed children in a population-based longitudinal follow-up study [45]. A case–control, blinded-evaluator study showed that phenytoin-exposed children had significantly lower IQ scores [57]. A prospective blinded observational study reported lower IQ for children with fetal phenytoin exposure compared with matched controls [44], although no effect was seen when maternal IQ was considered [58]. In a prospective observational multicenter study of monotherapy, children at age 3 who were exposed to phenytoin *in utero* had better IQ outcomes than those exposed to valproate but did not differ from those exposed to carbamazepine or lamotrigine [49]. Avoiding phenytoin in women with epilepsy during pregnancy is recommended by the American Academy of Neurology based on level C evidence [55]; however, firm conclusions on the risks of phenytoin require additional studies.

Valproate

Lower verbal IQ or full-scale IQ was demonstrated in children of women with epilepsy exposed *in utero* to valproate monotherapy compared to children with carbamazepine monotherapy in two prospective, population-based, evaluator-blinded studies [4,47]. However, the sample size of the valproate monotherapy group limited these studies ($N=26$ across the two studies). In addition, the studies showed significantly lower maternal education or IQ in the valproate group compared with other women with epilepsy. In another study of retrospective design, children exposed to valproate monotherapy had an increased need of special education compared with children exposed to other monotherapies or compared with an unexposed group [7]. In another study, lower verbal IQ (about 10 points) was seen in children exposed *in utero* to valproate ($N=41$) versus other monotherapy groups and versus an unexposed group. This was a large retrospective investigation that controlled for maternal IQ [46]. The decrease in IQ in the valproate group was a dose-dependent effect.

A large, prospective, observational, evaluator-blinded, multicenter study enrolled pregnant women with epilepsy on AED monotherapy and found that their children at age 3 had lower IQ (7–9 points) if exposed to valproate compared with three other AEDs (carbamazepine, lamotrigine, or phenytoin) [49]. Valproate's effect was dose-dependent. According to a follow-up analysis in the same study, verbal and nonverbal cognitive outcomes were reduced in children exposed *in utero* to valproate monotherapy versus carbamazepine, lamotrigine, and phenytoin. Again, the effect was dose-dependent, and the impact of the effect appeared greater in verbal than in nonverbal abilities [12]. A second follow-up analysis [50] in the same study in 4.5-year-old children exposed *in utero* to valproate again showed lower IQ (11–12 points) compared with other AEDs (carbamazepine, lamotrigine, or phenytoin). Again the effect was dose-dependent. It was determined that adverse cognitive effects of fetal valproate exposure persist to 4.5 years and are related to performances at earlier ages.

The Australian Pregnancy Register for Women with Epilepsy and Allied Disorders has conducted two studies on language function in children exposed to AEDs. The first study included 57 children and evaluated cognitive impact of *in utero* exposure to valproate monotherapy, polytherapy without valproate, or polytherapy with valproate in school-aged children using the fourth edition of the Wechsler Intelligence Scale for Children [59]. All groups had elevated frequencies of extremely low (<70) or borderline (70–79) full-scale IQ (15.8–40.0%). Working Memory scores and Verbal Comprehension were significantly below the standardized test mean in all groups. The results suggest that valproate may affect working memory and that it has a dose-dependent negative impact on verbal intellectual abilities. The second Australian study included 102 children exposed to AEDs [60]; language abilities were assessed using the Clinical Evaluation of Language Fundamental (CELF-4). Mean core language scores were carbamazepine monotherapy, 98.9; lamotrigine monotherapy, 106.3; valproate monotherapy, 91.5; polytherapy with valproate, 73.4; and polytherapy without valproate, 95.6 [60]. Exposure to valproate in monotherapy or polytherapy was associated with lower language scores. Valproate dose was negatively correlated with language scores.

An increased risk for autistic spectrum disorder or behavioral abnormalities in valproate-exposed children has been posited in two retrospective and one prospective study [48,61,62]. Avoiding valproate in women with epilepsy during pregnancy, if possible, should be considered to reduce the risk of poor cognitive and verbal outcomes (level B) [55].

Benzodiazepines

The risks of fetal exposure to benzodiazepines on cognition and behavior are largely unknown due to a lack of adequate data in human studies.

Other AEDs

The risks of fetal exposure to other AEDs on cognition and behavior are largely unknown due to a lack of adequate data in human studies.

Polytherapy

One prospective study published in 1976 reported no IQ difference between children exposed to phenytoin and phenobarbital polytherapy versus other children of women with epilepsy [52]. Subsequent prospective studies have found otherwise. Lower cognitive scores were seen in children exposed *in utero* to AED polytherapy versus healthy controls and children of women with epilepsy exposed to monotherapy [63]. Additional studies revealed impaired verbal and nonverbal IQ in children exposed *in utero* to AED polytherapy compared with children exposed to monotherapy alone [4,64]. If possible, AED polytherapy should be avoided in women with epilepsy to reduce the risk of poor cognitive and verbal outcomes.

Breastfeeding and AEDs

There is concern that breastfeeding during AED therapy may be harmful to cognitive development even though breastfeeding is known to be beneficial for the infant and mother [65]. In one investigation on cognitive outcomes at age 3 years in children previously exposed *in utero* to AEDs, breastfeeding during AED therapy failed to demonstrate deleterious effects (i.e., carbamazepine, lamotrigine, phenytoin, or valproate monotherapy). However, this was the only study of its kind and therefore additional research is needed to confirm this finding [66,67].

Conclusions on cognitive outcomes from human studies

From the current literature, the most prominent signal with respect to a specific AED is that fetal valproate exposure poses a special dose-dependent risk for cognitive development in the child. Valproate also carries the risk of anatomical teratogenesis in addition to the behavioral/cognitive risks. Carbamazepine and lamotrigine appear to have low risk for cognitive development based on current studies. The risks for many of the other AEDs are uncertain due to inadequate or inconsistent data. Polytherapy exposure also poses a special risk to cognitive development based on limited studies; however, the risks of specific AED combinations is unclear. A multitude of questions remain unanswered, and there is a critical need for future research.

Implications for management

Discussion of the risks and choice of AED should be done prior to pregnancy. The use of pre-conception folate is also recommended but the specific optimal dose is unclear. The typical dose used in practice is 0.4–4 mg daily. If possible, use AED monotherapy in the lowest effective dose. Avoid valproate if possible in women of childbearing potential. If unable to avoid valproate, then use the lowest dose possible. Consider avoiding phenobarbital and polytherapy during pregnancy. Monitor AED levels during pregnancy to correct for metabolic changes and avoid increased risk of convulsions [67].

Review of the case: Based on a single discharge from one EEG, the diagnosis underlying the convulsions could be localization-related epilepsy, but generalized epilepsy cannot be ruled out. Given the age of onset, it could be juvenile myoclonic epilepsy, but there was no history of myoclonic jerks. She recently failed conversion to lamotrigine monotherapy, but it should be noted that her lamotrigine level was in the low therapeutic range even though she is on valproate. When valproate was withdrawn, the lamotrigine level would have been even lower. The lamotrigine level should have been checked prior to valproate withdrawal, and adjusted upward prior to changing valproate, and then a further increase in lamotrigine may have been needed after cessation of valproate. Lorazepam therapy during this transition may be considered to reduce the risk of breakthrough seizures, but now that she is pregnant the lorazepam poses a risk to the fetus. AED choice and alterations should ideally be done prior to pregnancy. In fact, these issues need to be addressed when a woman of childbearing potential is first started on an AED because approximately half of all pregnancies are unplanned.

Now that the patient presents pregnant, choices are more complicated. Switching AEDs in pregnancy will expose the fetus to polytherapy, and it will be uncertain if the mother and fetus would be exposed to the adverse effects of convulsions. Lamotrigine or any other AED other than valproate may not control her seizures. Valproate is the most efficacious drug for primary generalized epilepsy, but it poses the greatest risk to the fetus for dose-dependent birth defects and cognitive problems. Although most women with primary generalized epilepsy can be controlled by other AEDs, there is a subgroup of these women that can only be controlled by valproate.

In consultation with the patient, the decision was made to stop lamotrigine and to continue valproate, checking the level monthly and adjusting the dose for changes in clearance during pregnancy in order to maintain a target level in the "subtherapeutic" range of 40–43 μg/dL, similar to the levels she had in the past which had controlled her seizures. She remained seizure-free throughout pregnancy, and gave birth to a healthy child. After pregnancy, she was converted to levetiracetam and tapered off valproate, remaining seizure-free.

 Key summary points

- The majority of children born to women with epilepsy are normal, but they are at increased risk for both anatomical and behavioral teratogenic deficits.
- Many factors contribute to neurodevelopmental deficits in children of women with epilepsy.
- Children exposed to more than four GTCS *in utero* may be at risk for lower cognitive abilities.

- AEDs during pregnancy may negatively impact cognition in infants of women with epilepsy.
- Possible mechanisms of functional/behavioral teratogenicity from AED exposure include folate, reactive intermediates, ischemia, apoptosis, neuronal suppression, and alterations to neurotransmitter systems.
- Of the AEDs, valproate and polytherapy pose special risks and should be avoided if possible.
- Breastfeeding while mothers are taking AEDs appears to be safe based on limited data, but more research is needed.

References

1 Leavitt AM, Yerby MS, Robinson N, *et al.* Epilepsy in pregnancy: developmental outcome of offspring at 12 months. *Neurology* 1992;42(Suppl 5):141–143.
2 Yerby MS. Pregnancy and epilepsy. *Epilepsia.* 1991;32(Suppl 6):S51–S59.
3 Meador KJ. Cognitive effects of epilepsy and of antiepileptic medications. In: Wyllie E, Cascino GD, Gidal BE, Goodkin HP (eds) *The Treatment of Epilepsy: Principles and Practice,* 5th edn. Philadelphia: Lippincott Williams & Wilkins, 2011:1028–1036.
4 Gaily E, Kantola-Sorsa E, Hiilesmaa V *et al.* Normal intelligence in children with prenatal exposure to carbamazepine. *Neurology* 2004;62:28–32.
5 Holmes LB, Rosenberger PB, Harvey EA, Khoshbin S, Ryan L. Intelligence and physical features of children of women with epilepsy. *Teratology* 2000;61:196–202.
6 Gaily E, Kantola-Sorsa E, Granstrom ML. Intelligence of children of epileptic mothers. *J Pediatr* 1988;113:677–684.
7 Adab N, Jacoby A, Smith D, Chadwick D. Additional educational needs in children born to mothers with epilepsy. *J Neurol Neurosurg Psychiatry* 2001;70:15–21.
8 Hiilesmaa V. Effects of maternal seizures on the fetus. In: Tomson T, Gram L, Sillanpää M, Johannesen S (eds) *Epilepsy and Pregnancy.* Petersfield, UK and Bristol, PA, USA: Wrightson Biomedical Publishing Ltd, 1996:135–141.
9 Palac S, Meador KJ. Antiepileptic drugs and neurodevelopment: an update. *Curr Neurol Neurosci Rep* 2011;11:423–427.
10 Meador KJ, Reynolds RW, Crean S, Fahrbach K, Probst C. Pregnancy outcomes in women with epilepsy: a systematic review and meta-analysis of published pregnancy registries and cohorts. *Epilepsy Res* 2008;81:1–13.
11 Thomas SV, Sukumaran S, Lukose N, George A, Sarma PS. Intellectural and language functions in children of mothers with epilepsy. *Epilepsia* 2007;48:2234–2240.
12 Meador KJ, Baker GA, Browning N *et al.* Foetal antiepileptic drug exposure and verbal versus non-verbal abilities at three years of age. *Brain* 2011;134:396–404.
13 Adams J, Vorhees CV, Middaugh LD. Developmental neurotoxicity of anticonvulsants: human and animal evidence on phenytoin. *Neurotoxicol Teratol* 1990;12:203–214.
14 Fisher JE, Vorhees C. Developmental toxicity of antiepileptic drugs: relationship to postnatal dysfunction. *Pharmacol Res* 1992;26:207–221.
15 Meador KJ. Cognitive effects of epilepsy and of antiepileptic medications. In: Wyllie E (ed.) *The Treatment of Epilepsy. Principles and Practices,* 4th edn. Philadelphia: Lippincott Williams & Wilkins, 2005: 1185–1195.
16 Finnell RH, Chernoff GF. Gene–teratogen interactions. An approach to understanding the metabolic basis of birth defects. In: Nau H, Scott WJ (eds) *Pharmacokinetics in Teratogenesis.* Boca Raton, FL: CRC Press, 1987:97–109.

17 Phelan MC, Pellock JM, Nance WE. Discordant expression of fetal hydantoin syndrome in heteropaternal dizygotic twins. *N Engl J Med* 1982;307:99–101.

18 Buehler BA, Delimont D, van Waes M, Finnell RH. Prenatal prediction of risk of the fetal hydantoin syndrome. *N Engl J Med* 1990;322:1567–1572.

19 Wells PG, Zubovits JT, Wong ST, Molinari LM, Ali S. Modulation of phenytoin teratogenicity and embryonic covalent binding by acetylsalicylic acid, caffeic acid, and alpha-phenyl-*N-t*-butylnitrone: implications for bioactivation by prostaglandin synthetase. *Toxicol Appl Pharmacol* 1989;97:192–202.

20 Wells PG, Kim PM, Laposa RR, Nicol CJ, Parman T, Winn LM. Oxidative damage in chemical teratogenesis. *Mutat Res* 1997;396:65–78.

21 Wong M, Wells PG. Modulation of embryonic glutathione reductase and phenytoin teratogenicity by 1,3-bis(2-chloroethyl)-1-nitrosourea (BCNU). *J Pharmacol Exp Ther* 1989;250:336–342.

22 Danielsson B, Sköld AC, Azarbayjani F, Ohman I, Webster W. Pharmacokinetic data support pharmacologically induced embryonic dysrhythmia as explanation to fetal hydantoin syndrome in rats. *Toxicol Appl Pharmacol* 2000;163:164–175.

23 Carl GF, Smith DB. Interaction of phenytoin and folate in the rat. *Epilepsia* 1983;24:494–501.

24 Carl GF, Smith DB. Effect of chronic phenobarbital treatment on folates and one-carbon enzymes in the rat. *Biochem Pharmacol* 1984;21:3457–3463.

25 Carl GF, Smith ML. Chronic primidone treatment in the rat: an animal model of primidone therapy. *Res Commun Chem Pathol Pharmacol* 1988;61:365–376.

26 Carl GF, Smith ML. Chronic carbamazepine treatment in the rat: efficacy, toxicity, and effect on plasma and tissue folate concentrations. *Epilepsia* 1989;30:217–224.

27 Carl GF, DeLoach C, Patterson J. Chronic sodium valproate treatment in the rat: toxicity versus protection against seizures induced by Indoklon. *Neurochem Int* 1986;8:41–45.

28 Danksy LV, Andermann E, Rosenblatt D, Sherwin AL, Andermann F. Anticonvulsants, folate levels and pregnancy outcome: a prospective study. *Ann Neurol* 1987;21:176–182.

29 Biale Y, Lewenthal H. Effect of folic acid supplementation on congenital malformations due to anticonvulsant drugs. *Eur J Obstet Gynecol Reprod Biol* 1984;18:211–216.

30 Ikonomidou C, Bittigau P, Ishimaru MJ *et al.* Ethanol-induced apoptotic neurodegeneration in fetal alcohol syndrome. *Science* 2000;287:1056–1060.

31 Medina AE, Krahe TE, Coppola DM, Ramoa AS. Neonatal alcohol exposure induces long-lasting impairment of visual cortical plasticity in ferrets. *J Neurosci* 2003;23:10002–10012.

32 Bittigau P, Sifringer M, Genz K *et al.* Antiepileptic drugs and apoptotic neurodegeneration in the developing brain. *Proc Natl Acad Sci USA* 2002;99:15089–15094.

33 Bittigau P, Sifringer M, Ikonomidou C. Antiepileptic drugs and apoptosis in the developing brain. *Ann NY Acad Sci* 2003;993:103–114; discussion 123–124.

34 Asimiadou S, Bittigau P, Felderhoff-Mueser U *et al.* Protection with estradiol in developmental models of apoptotic neurodegeneration. *Ann Neurol* 2005;58:266–276.

35 Stefovska VG, Uckermann O, Czuczwar M *et al.* Sedative and anticonvulsant drugs suppress postnatal neurogenesis. *Ann Neurol* 2008;64:434–445.

36 Ikonomidou C, Turski L. Antiepileptic drugs and brain development. *Epilepsy Res* 2010;88:11–22.

37 Katz I, Kim J, Gale K, Kondratyev A. Effects of lamotrigine alone and in combination with MK-801, phenobarbital, or phenytoin on cell death in the neonatal rat brain. *J Pharmacol Exp Ther* 2007;322:494–500.

38 Glier C, Dzietko M, Bittigau P, Jarosz B, Korobowicz E, Ikonomidou C. Therapeutic doses of topiramate are not toxic to the developing rat brain. *Exp Neurol* 2004;187:403–409.

39 Manthey D, Asimiadou S, Stefovska V *et al.* Sulthiame but not levetiracetam exerts neurotoxic effect in the developing rat brain. *Exp Neurol* 2005;193:497–503.

40 Kim J, Kondratyev A, Gale K. Antiepileptic drug-induced neuronal cell death in the immature brain: effects of carbamazepine, topiramate, and levetiracetam as monotherapy versus polytherapy. *J Pharmacol Exp Ther* 2007;323:165–173.

41 Manent JB, Jorquera I, Mazzucchelli I *et al.* Fetal exposure to GABA-acting antiepileptic drugs generates hippocampal and cortical dysplasias. *Epilepsia* 2007;48:684–693.

42 Wong WT, Wong RO. Changing specificity of neurotransmitter regulation of rapid dendritic remodeling during synaptogenesis. *Nat Neurosci* 2001;4:351–352.

43 Ogura H, Yasuda M, Nakamura S, Yamashita H, Mikoshiba K, Ohmori H. Neurotoxic damage of granule cells in the dentate gyrus and the cerebellum and cognitive deficit following neonatal administration of phenytoin in mice. *J Neuropathol Exp Neurol* 2002;61:956–967.

44 Scolnik D, Nulman I, Rovet J *et al.* Neurodevelopment of children exposed in utero to phenytoin and carbamazepine monotherapy. *JAMA* 1994;271:767–770.

45 Wide K, Hening E, Tomson T, Winbladh B. Psychomotor development in preschool children exposed to antiepileptic drugs in utero. *Acta Paediatr* 2002;91:409–414.

46 Adab N, Kini U, Vinten J *et al.* The longer term outcome of children born to mothers with epilepsy. *J Neurol Neurosurg Psychiatry* 2004;75:1575–1583.

47 Eriksson K, Viinikainen K, Mönkkönen A *et al.* Children exposed to valproate in utero: population based evaluation of risks and confounding factors for long-term neurocognitive development. *Epilepsy Res* 2005;65:189–200.

48 Rasalam AD, Hailey H, Williams LHG *et al.* Characteristics of fetal anticonvulsant syndrome associated autistic disorder. *Dev Med Child Neurol* 2005;47:551–555.

49 Meador KJ, Baker GA, Browning N *et al.* Fetal antiepileptic drug exposure and cognitive function at age 3. *N Engl J Med* 2009;360:1597–1605.

50 Meador KJ, Baker GA, Browning N *et al.* Effects of fetal antiepileptic drug exposure: outcomes at age 4.5 years. Neurology 2012;78:1207–1214.

51 Shallcross R, Bromley RL, Irwin B, Bonnett LJ, Morrow J, Baker GA. Liverpool Manchester Neurodevelopment Group; UK Epilepsy and Pregnancy Register. Child development following in utero exposure: levetiracetam vs. sodium valproate. *Neurology* 2011;76:383–399.

52 Shapiro S, Hartz SC, Siskind V *et al.* Anticonvulsants and parental epilepsy in the development of birth defects. *Lancet* 1976;i:272–275.

53 Reinisch JM, Sanders SA, Mortensen EL, Rubin DB. In utero exposure to phenobarbital and intelligence deficits in adult men. *JAMA* 1995;274:1518–1525.

54 Farwell JR, Young JL, Hirtz DG, Sulzbacher SI, Ellenberg JH, Nelson KB. Phenobarbital for febrile seizures: effects on intelligence and on seizure recurrence. *N Engl J Med* 1990;322:364–369.

55 Harden CL, Meador KJ, Pennell PB, Hauser WA, Gronseth GS, French JA. Practice parameter update: management issues for women with epilepsy. Focus on pregnancy (an evidence-based review): teratogenesis and perinatal outcomes. Report of the Quality Standards Subcommittee and Therapeutics and Technology Subcommittee of the American Academy of Neurology and American Epilepsy Society. *Neurology* 2009;73:133–141.

56 Hanson JW, Myrianthopoulos NC, Harvey MA, Smith DW. Risks to the offspring of women treated with hydantoin anticonvulsants, with emphasis on the fetal hydantoin syndrome. *J Pediatr* 1976;89:662–668.

57 Vanoverloop D, Schnell RR, Harvey EA, Holmes LB. The effects of prenatal exposure to phenytoin and other anticonvulsants on intellectual function at 4 to 8 years of age. *Neurotoxicol Teratol* 1992;14:329–335.

58 Loring DW, Meador KJ, Thompson WO. Neurodevelopment effects of phenytoin and carbamazepine. *JAMA* 1994;272:850–851.

59 Nadebaum C, Anderson V, Vajda F, Reutens D, Barton S, Wood A. The Australian Brain and Cognition and Antiepileptic Drugs Study: IQ in school-aged children exposed to sodium valproate and polytherapy. *J Int Neuropsychol Soc* 2011;17: 133–142.

60 Nadebaum C, Anderson VA, Vajda F, Reutens DC, Barton S, Wood AG. Language skills of school-aged children prenatally exposed to antiepileptic drugs. *Neurology* 2011;76:719–726.

61 Bromley RL, Mawer G, Clayton-Smith J, Baker GA. Autism spectrum disorders following in utero exposure to antiepileptic drugs. *Neurology* 2008;71:1923–1924.

62 Vinten J, Bromley RL, Taylor J, Adab N, Kini U, Baker GA. The behavioral consequences of exposure to antiepileptic drugs in utero. *Epilepsy Behav* 2009;14: 197–201.

63 Lösche G, Steinhausen HC, Koch S, Helge H. The psychological development of children of epileptic parents. II. The differential impact of intrauterine exposure to anticonvulsant drugs and further influential factors. *Acta Paediatr* 1994;83:961–966.

64 Koch S, Titze K, Zimmermann RB, Schröder M, Lehmkuhl U, Rauh H. Long-term neuropsychological consequences of maternal epilepsy and anticonvulsant treatment during pregnancy for school-age children and adolescents. *Epilepsia* 1999;40:1237–1243.

65 Ip S, Chung M, Raman G *et al.* A summary of the Agency for Healthcare Research and Quality's evidence report on breast-feeding in developed countries. *Breastfeed Med* 2009;4(Suppl 1):S17–S30.

66 Meador KJ, Baker GA, Browning N *et al.* Effects of breast-feeding in children of women on antiepileptic drugs. *Neurology* 2010;75:1954–1960.

67 Meador KJ. Neurodevelopmental impact of antiepileptic drugs. In: Helmstaedter C, Hermann G, Lassonde M, Kahane P, Arzimanoglou A (eds) *Neuropsychology in the Care of People with Epilepsy*. Progress in Epileptic Disorders Vol. 11. Montrouge, France: Editions John Libby Eurotext, 2011.

CHAPTER 16

Management of the Postpartum Period and Lactation

Autumn M. Klein

Departments of Neurology and Obstetrics and Gynecology, UPMC Presbyterian/Magee Women's Hospital of UPMC, Pittsburgh, Pennsylvania, USA

> **Case history:** *L.B. is a 39-year-old G1P1 who has had seizures since the age of 15 and has just vaginally delivered a healthy baby boy at 39 weeks after spontaneous labor. The patient describes her seizures as nausea and déjà vu followed by loss of consciousness and automatisms, accompanied by blinking and staring without clear lateralized movements. She will walk away from events or activities during the seizure and often finds herself in corners, doorways, or under a tree and has a few minutes of confusion after her seizures. Triggers are significant lack of sleep, intense physical exercise, and her menstrual period. Approximately once every few years she has a secondarily generalized convulsion. She has been on many medications, including carbamazepine, phenytoin, valproic acid, oxcarbazepine and, most recently, at the age of 35 when contemplating marriage and children, was switched to lamotrigine. Levetiracetam was then added, resulting in optimal control. She attained her best seizure control thus far with this latest medication combination. She continued to have four to five complex partial seizures a month and a convulsion once every few years, the most recent occurring 5 months prior to conception of this pregnancy. She has left mesial temporal sclerosis and video-EEG has captured all seizures arising from this location, but she has refused surgical evaluation. She did quite well throughout the pregnancy and delivery with serum antiepileptic drug (AED) monitoring and she wants to breastfeed.*

Breastfeeding: background and benefits

The World Alliance for Breastfeeding Action has a mission to protect, promote, and support breastfeeding worldwide. The health benefits of breastfeeding for mothers and children are clear, yet the practice is far from universally adopted. For example, in the USA the 2011 Breastfeeding Report Card showed that, overall, 74.6% of women have ever breastfed, with 44.3% and 23.8% of women breastfeeding at 6 and 12 months, respectively. Only 35% and 14.8% of women were exclusively breastfeeding at 3 and

---

Epilepsy in Women, First Edition. Edited by Cynthia L. Harden, Sanjeev V. Thomas and Torbjörn Tomson.

6 months, respectively [1]. The rate of women with epilepsy (WWE) who are breastfeeding is not clearly known. In one recent study which enrolled mostly educated white women, 42% of WWE were breastfeeding [2].

Breastfeeding has been shown to have numerous short- and long-term health benefits for mothers and also for infant health, growth, immunity, and development [3,4]. In a meta-analysis published by the Agency for Research and Quality, breastfeeding decreases a woman's risk of developing diabetes and breast and ovarian cancers, while in infants it reduces the risk of ear infections, diarrheal illnesses, asthma, obesity, sudden infant death syndrome, and leukemia [3]. It also promotes mother–infant attachment and is psychologically beneficial to both mother and child.

Many psychosocial factors are known to influence whether a mother breastfeeds, including her initial determination, the time she has with the child (i.e., whether or not she returns to work), and the personal support from her family, workplace, and healthcare system. For many women, breastfeeding can be difficult to initiate due to difficulties with the child latching on and sucking, resulting in sore or painful nipples. Many birthing hospitals do not have a full complement of lactation consultants, thereby limiting education on breastfeeding, and with many women going home within 2–4 days after birth without other supportive family at home, the resources for continuing teaching are further limited.

Women with epilepsy and breastfeeding

Despite all the support and the known benefits of breastfeeding, many WWE are still hesitant to breastfeed their children but the reasons are not entirely clear. Concerns include their psychosocial situation, the severity of the disease, the AEDs needed to control seizures, the effects of breastfeeding on seizures, and the effects of seizures on breastfeeding. When the developing offspring is *in utero*, many WWE must remain on AEDs for seizure control and so the child is exposed to the AEDs through the maternal circulation and the placenta. Once the child is born, AED exposure through breast milk is voluntary and at the choice of the parents. Many women do not understand the amount of drug that the child experiences through breast milk, and some think that the child experiences *more* drug through breast milk than *in utero*. While all AEDs can pass into breast milk, the amount transferred into breast milk is almost always less than the amount transmitted through the placenta. For many AEDs, though, the amounts getting into the breast milk are unknown.

Many factors influence the amount of drug that gets into breast milk, and this is dependent on drug properties as well as maternal and newborn physiology. While the amount in breast milk is important, ultimately what the child extracts from the breast milk is physiologically the most critical value. Medications themselves have different properties that influence whether or not they get into the breast milk, including molecular size, pH, and protein binding. Other factors include the frequency of dosing, the time from drug administration to the time of breast milk sampling, where the sample is drawn from (foremilk, hindmilk, breast side), the frequency of nursing, the length of lactation, and the degree of lactation (exclusively breastfeeding or bottle and breastfeeding). Frequent sampling is ideal for obtaining an accurate level, but most of the time only one sample is obtained. Unfortunately, much of the current literature is obtained from older studies when pharmacokinetic techniques were not as sensitive and from samples obtained from mothers who were not "allowed" to breast-feed. Animal models are not helpful since breast milk composition is quite different in humans.

There are presumed effects of AEDs on long-term child development and behavior, but it is not entirely clear if there is a short-term perinatal AED withdrawal syndrome. With some AEDs this is a greater concern, but in general there are rare reports of symptoms that may be interpreted as withdrawal. These include sedation, lethargy, irritability, excessive crying, altered sleep patterns, vomiting, difficulty feeding, and tremor. Some children exposed to barbiturates at high levels experience withdrawal and need continued observation, but this is not always the case. The concern with this is highest with primidone and phenobarbital. Breastfeeding may ameliorate these withdrawal symptoms as the child is experiencing less medication over time [5]. There are no well-established standards for measuring withdrawal in neonates, making comparisons to the general population difficult. Additionally, offspring of WWE taking AEDs may be under greater scrutiny than most neonates, thereby leading to an observation bias.

Ultimately, the best determination of drug effect is the offspring's serum level, which can be done via heelstick to avoid venipuncture. This is the most accurate and reassuring way to assess drug exposure in the child. Most reported adverse effects of drugs in breast milk are seen in children less than 6 months of age, which coincides with the time frame that most women breastfeed. Based on a study of different classes of drugs, including antiepileptics, when the baby's serum level is less than 10% of the mother's serum level, then it is felt to be clinically insignificant [6]. Levels higher than this are not a contraindication to breastfeeding, but a risk–benefit analysis should be discussed with the patient.

Neonatal factors also affect breastfeeding ability and drug exposure. It is thought that more infants born to WWE are preterm or premature, making breastfeeding more difficult if their suck and swallow is less developed. Some medications may make the child initially more sedated, further slowing their ability to begin proper feeding within the first few days of life. Premature children and children who are small for gestational age may be less efficient at extracting medications from breast milk. Additionally, metabolism of medications is slower in infants than in adults, thereby prolonging their half-life and excretion. As the child gets older, they are more able to extract nutrients from their food and their metabolism of medications increases.

It is known that the UDP-glucuronyltransferase (UGT) enzymes that metabolize many medications, including lamotrigine, have low activity at birth but increase to the adult level at around 20 months of age [7]. While levels of AEDs like lamotrigine have been shown to be much lower than maternal serum levels, but metabolism and elimination are still slowed [8]. In general, it is felt that there are no significant adverse effects associated with breastfeeding and lamotrigine, but there is one reported case of apnea in an infant who was exclusively breastfed and whose mother was taking lamotrigine [9]. Other factors that are known to significantly alter rates of drug metabolism, such as genetic polymorphisms, have not been studied in the metabolism of AEDs in infants.

While this chapter does not focus on AED adjustment in the pregnant and postpartum mother, many AEDs are increased during pregnancy and then usually decreased at some point in the postpartum period. Many factors are involved in determining when these adjustments occur, but many epileptologists make these changes depending on the drug, the relative pre-pregnancy dose, and the postpartum seizure risk. Most patients at delivery are on doses higher than they were before pregnancy, thereby increasing the risk of postpartum toxicity, particularly with lamotrigine. This not only increases the amount of medication that may get into the breast milk, but also increases the risk that the mother may experience toxic side effects after birth, thereby limiting her ability to care for her child.

Breastfeeding guidelines

In medical situations of uncertainty, guidelines are useful to help with decisions. The American Academy of Neurology (AAN) and the American Academy of Pediatrics (AAP) have addressed some of the concerns related to AEDs and breastfeeding.

The AAN practice parameters concluded that primidone and levetiracetam penetrate into breast milk in potentially clinically important amounts [10]. They also noted that valproate, phenobarbital, phenytoin, and carbamazepine probably do not pass into breast milk in clinically significant quantities, and that gabapentin, lamotrigine, and topiramate possibly get into breast milk in potentially clinically significant amounts. Their final statement was that "the clinical consequences for the newborn of ingesting AEDs via breast milk remain sorely underexplored and will continue to produce anxiety in WWE bearing children and all who care for these clinical dyads" [10]. Despite the lack of information on AEDs in breast milk, in general, for most AEDs, many epileptologists feel that the benefits of breastfeeding probably outweigh the risks of AED exposure.

This risk–benefit balance should be more carefully evaluated with barbiturates and benzodiazepines. While levels of phenobarbital and primidone are low in breast milk, it is generally not recommended to breastfeed while taking either due to reports of sedation and serum levels that are higher in the child than in the mother [11]. The AAP suggests administering with caution [12]. It has also been shown that children breastfed while mother was taking diazepam had lethargy, weight loss, and sedation. The AAP states that the effects in breastfeeding are unknown and to exercise caution [12].

Most medications show low transfer into breast milk. Medications with higher protein binding (carbamazepine, phenytoin, valproate) show little transfer into breast milk and it is for this reason that the AAP recommends that these medications are compatible with breastfeeding [12]. Despite the great interest in breastfeeding, there are very few reports of AED levels in breast milk and infant serum. Where information is available, evidence on AEDs used more commonly in reproductive-age women is presented briefly in the following sections.

Valproic acid

Valproic acid was studied in the breast milk of six mother–infant pairs and the levels in the infants were shown to be 0.9–2.3% of mother's serum level [13]. A similar study showed that two infant's serum levels of valproate were 1.5 and 6.0% [14]. Older studies using drug levels measured by mass spectroscopy analysis in 36 breast milk samples from 16 patients showed that the range of valproate levels was also very low at 0.4–3.9 µg/mL (mean 1.9 ± 1.2 µg/mL) [15]. Interestingly, they also showed that the total and free levels in breast milk were similar. There is only one known adverse report of an infant who had thrombocytopenia and anemia while being breastfed on valproate [16].

Phenytoin

There have been no recent studies on the levels of phenytoin in breast milk. It has been shown that in infants of mothers taking phenytoin there are very low levels of phenytoin in the serum (<5% of maternal serum) [17]. There was one report in 1954 of methemaglobinemia, drowsiness, and decreased suck in one infant breastfed on phenytoin [18], but no adverse reports recently.

Carbamazepine

Levels of carbamazepine are low in breast milk and infants, with milk/maternal serum ratios of 0.64 and 0.3 in two infants [19]. This is similar to other reported cases. Another older study showed that the carbamazepine concentration in breast milk was 36.4% of the maternal carbamazepine serum level but the authors did not measure infant serum [20]. There have been two reports of liver dysfunction and hepatitis from carbamazepine administration during pregnancy and after birth [21].

Lamotrigine

The largest case series of lamotrigine in breast milk studied 30 women and their infants, with 210 samples of breast milk [22]. The milk to maternal plasma ratio was 41.3%, with an infant serum dose 18.9% that of the maternal serum dose. Only mild thrombocytopenia was noted in the children. A previous report that studied nine women on lamotrigine monotherapy found a milk to maternal serum ratio of 0.59 (range 0.35–0.86) [23]. Another study with four mothers on lamotrigine monotherapy showed that newborn levels were 30% of maternal serum levels, but this did not decline after 2 months [8]. Previous studies showed similar findings in smaller groups of mother–child pairs [24].

There is one case report of a child exposed to lamotrigine through full breastfeeding and who had an episode of apnea. While the authors suggest there is a correlation, the child had a lower level of lamotrigine at the time of the apnea 16 days after birth (4.87 µg/mL) than he did at 12.5 hours after birth (7.71 µg/mL) [9].

Levetiracetam

In a recent study of 11 mothers who breastfed and gave breast milk and infant serum samples, the average milk/maternal serum ratio was 1.05 (range 0.78–1.55) and the infant's level was 13% of the mother's serum level [25]. This suggests that while transfer to breast milk is high, the amount the infant absorbs is low. Another study followed eight mothers and their infants from birth to 10 months of age [26]. At 3–5 days, milk/maternal serum level was 1.00 (range 0.76–1.33) and infant serum levels were very low at 10–15 µmol/L. These findings were stable at all later time points.

Topiramate

Breast milk information on five mother–child pairs showed milk/maternal plasma ratio was 0.86 (range 0.67–1.1) at 2–3 weeks after delivery and was similar again at 1 and 3 months after birth [27]. Two to three weeks after delivery, infants had barely detectable levels (>0.9 µmol/L) that could not be quantified and one had undetectable levels. There are no clear adverse events related to breastfeeding a child on topiramate.

Zonisamide

In two mothers taking zonismade, 41–57% of the drug was excreted into the breast milk [28]. There are no reports of adverse events in an infant exposed to zonisamide through breast milk.

Other AEDs

There are no known reports of breastfeeding with lacosamide, pregabalin, retigabine, rufinamide, tiagabine, or vigabatrin. It is evident from this review that there is very little information on AEDs and breastfeeding and more needs to be done.

While there is no consensus, and this is not addressed in any guidelines, it would generally not be recommended to start an AED after birth while breastfeeding since the offspring was not exposed to an AED *in utero*.

Effects on cognition in offspring exposed to AEDs through breastfeeding

There is little information on the cognitive and behavioral outcomes of children born to mothers taking AEDs and breastfeeding. In the Neurocognitive Effects of Antiepileptic Drugs (NEAD) study, the offspring of WWE taking monotherapy of carbamazepine, lamotrigine, phenytoin, or valproate were studied according to drug and breastfeeding status and whether those who breastfed on a particular drug differed from those who did not breastfeed on the same drug [2]. Overall and for each specific drug, there was no difference between those children who were breastfed and those who were not breastfed at the 3-year IQ testing, suggesting that breastfeeding does not have a harmful effect on cognition. More studies need to be done to determine these long-term effects.

Safety issues

Once a child is born, the mother often neglects her own health and well-being. New mothers focus on the care of the infant and may forget their own medical and personal needs (i.e., medications, sleep) and how that influences the care of their child. The postpartum period is a difficult time both physically and emotionally, and WWE are particularly vulnerable during this time. There has been very little in the literature on postpartum safety in WWE. In one study WWE who used Epilepsy Action in the UK answered a questionnaire about the risks of caring for their baby and the information that they were given on this [29]. Mothers stated that they were most concerned about caring for their baby outside the home and bathing them as compared with breastfeeding. Almost 50% of them had been given information on safety and 86% stated that they found it useful. Postpartum safety certainly deserves more attention.

Sleep deprivation is a hallmark of the postpartum period for any mother but this is of great concern for WWE. Since lack of sleep is a known seizure trigger, this is a particularly difficult time for WWE in caring for their child. It is ideal if WWE can arrange for family or hired help to assist with night-time wakenings and feedings. Breastfed babies usually need more frequent feedings (on average, once every 2–3 hours instead of once every 4–5 hours) and so many WWE must balance sleep with feeding at the breast. Milk that is pumped in advance can be fed to the baby, but there is still the need to pump frequently to maintain milk supply.

It is important to review day-to-day activities to ensure that mother and child are safe should a seizure occur. Considering the seizure type and whether there is a warning is critical to planning safe practices for mother and child. For the mother with an aura or warning, it is suggested that she places the baby in a crib or other enclosed safe space as soon as the warning occurs. For mothers with jerks from myoclonic seizures, ensuring good sleep is the best way to avoid the myoclonus; knowing the critical periods when these might occur (i.e., in the morning) helps to determine when not to hold the child. In some cases, particularly if mother has no warning or has convulsive seizures, having family or other caregivers around as much as possible is ideal. Bathing a child or breastfeeding the child in bed when the mother is alone is not recommended. Any activities, such as changing the baby or playing with the child, are best done on a rug or as close to the ground as possible in case the mother has to lay down or falls down during a seizure.

When children get older and start to crawl or walk, keeping them in a safe enclosed area is suggested; if the mother has a seizure, the child will not be put in danger by wandering off or getting into dangerous situations. For mothers taking children outside the home, safe practices should be reviewed in advance and an emergency plan devised. Going to a playground or a public place where there are other families with children or going to locations where those around are aware that the mother has epilepsy is suggested. In some cases, it may be helpful for the child to wear a Medic Alert bracelet or to pin a message to the child with instructions such as who to call or what to do in the event mother has a seizure. Investigating epilepsy support groups that offer meetings for mothers to discuss their concerns and plans for safety are helpful for WWE and can reduce their concerns over these situations.

Depression

Postpartum depression (PPD) is characterized by mood swings, irritability, tearfulness, fatigue and confusion, occurs in the first few weeks after birth, and is usually transient. It affects on average about 15% of women, but women with depression prior to pregnancy are at increased risk [30]. Ideal treatments are psychotherapy followed by antidepressants, but many women cannot adequately access psychotherapy in the postpartum period and/or are hesitant to take psychoactive medications while breastfeeding.

As for many women with chronic disease, the rates of PPD have been shown to be higher in WWE compared with the general population [31, 32]. One study administered the Edinburgh Postnatal Depression Scale in WWE and healthy controls and found that 29% of WWE had PPD compared with only 11% of controls. In another study administering the Beck Depression Inventory in 56 WWE during pregnancy and after birth, 25% of women were shown to have PPD that appeared to be associated with multiparity and AED polytherapy but unrelated to a specific AED [32]. There are many reasons why WWE are at increased risk of PPD. In addition to the fact that WWE have a higher rate of depression than the general population, their interactions with the baby may be limited due to their concerns about seizures and holding the baby, limited mobility and social interaction due to inability to drive, and more monetary constraints than women without epilepsy. These are all concerns that also add to anxiety and worry for the mother. WWE need reassurance and support from their physician and family to help offset their concerns. Being aware of the increased risks of PPD for WWE can help identify it earlier and get treatment faster.

Contraception in the immediate postpartum period

Discussing future family planning during pregnancy may prevent unintended pregnancies. There are still many women, particularly adolescents and young mothers, who believe that they cannot get pregnant while breastfeeding or during the postpartum period. While this is beyond the scope of this chapter and discussed elsewhere in this book, contraceptive options such as tubal ligation or medroxyprogesterone injections can be started immediately after birth and help to avoid delay.

Implications for management

The postpartum period is a very challenging time for many new mothers, but for WWE there are added considerations about breastfeeding, depression, and safety. Discussing information about the AED and the amount that gets into the breast milk and child is paramount to ensuring the best choice is made for the mother and child. Making the husband and family aware that WWE are at increased risk of depression, particularly if they have had a personal history of depression, can avert major depressive episodes and help women get treatment faster. Finally, patient and child safety is one of the greatest postpartum concerns WWE have. Addressing this with the mother and family in advance of the birth will help them prepare for special house arrangements and extra help where needed. Planning ahead, educating the patient and family about these issues, and making regular follow-up appointments in the postpartum period can help avoid seizures and injury or harm to the newborn.

Review of the case: L.B. breastfed exclusively for almost 1 year. Her seizures continued to remain under good control and her child met all milestones and there were no concerns raised by the pediatrician. She and her husband worked out a schedule so she could sleep six uninterrupted hours every night and she napped with the baby every day for 2–3 hours. She never bathed the baby alone and put him in a crib when she had an aura. If she had an aura outside, she would clip the baby's stroller to her wrist with a short chain and kept contact information in a visible pocket on the outside of the stroller. Mother and child did well without injury.

 Key summary points
- Breastfeeding is encouraged in WWE.
- WWE are concerned about caring for their newborn infant. Advanced planning can decrease risk of injury to mother and newborn.
- WWE are at increased risk of postpartum depression. Early awareness can lead to faster treatment.
- Discuss postpartum contraception during pregnancy.

References

1 Centers for Disease Control and Prevention. Breastfeeding Report Card, United States, 2011. Available at www.cdc.gov/breastfeeding/pdf/2011breastfeedingreportcard.pdf
2 Meador KJ, Baker GA, Browning N *et al.* Effects of breastfeeding in children of women taking antiepileptic drugs. *Neurology* 2010;75:1954–1960.
3 Agency for Healthcare Research and Quality. Breastfeeding and maternal and infant health outcomes in developed countries [updated April 2007]. Available at www.ahrq.gov/clinic/tp/brfouttp.htm
4 American Academy of Pediatrics Section on Breastfeeding. Breastfeeding and the use of human milk. *Pediatrics* 2005;115:496–506.
5 Rauchenzauner M, Kiechl-Kohlendorfer U, Rostasy K, Luef G. Old and new antiepileptic drugs during pregnancy and lactation: report of a case. *Epilepsy Behav* 2011;20:719–720.
6 Ito, S. Drug therapy for breast-feeding women. *N Engl J Med* 2000;343:118–126.

7 Miyagi SJ, Collier AC. Pediatric development of glucuronidation: the ontogeny of hepatic UGT1A4. *Drug Metab Dispos* 2007;35:1587–1592.

8 Liporace J, Kao A, D'Abreu A. Concerns regarding lamotrigine and breast-feeding. *Epilepsy Behav* 2004;5:102–105.

9 Nordmo E, Aronsen L, Wasland K, Smabrekke L, Vorren S. Severe apnea in an infant exposed to lamotrigine in breast milk. *Ann Pharmacother* 2009;43:1893–1897.

10 Harden CL, Pennell PB, Koppel BS *et al.* Practice parameter update: management issues for women with epilepsy. Focus on pregnancy (an evidence-based review): vitamin K, folic acid, blood levels, and breastfeeding: report of the Quality Standards Subcommittee and Therapeutics and Technology Assessment Subcommittee of the American Academy of Neurology and American Epilepsy Society. *Neurology* 2009;73:142–149.

11 Kaneko S, Sato T, Suzuki K. The levels of anticonvulsants in breast milk. *Br J Clin Pharmacol* 1979;7:624–627.

12 American Academy of Pediatrics Committee on Drugs. Transfer of drugs and other chemicals into human milk. *Pediatrics* 2001;108:776–789.

13 Piontek CM, Baab S, Peindl KS, Wisner KL. Serum valproate levels in 6 breastfeeding mother–infant pairs. *J Clin Psychiatry* 2000;61:170–172.

14 Wisner KL, Perel JM. Serum levels of valproate and carbamazepine in breastfeeding mother–infant pairs. *J Clin Psychopharmacol* 1998;18:167–169.

15 von Unruh GE, Froescher W, Hoffmann F, Niesen M. Valproic acid in breast milk: how much is really there? *Ther Drug Monit* 1984;6:272–276.

16 Stahl MM, Neiderud J, Vinge E. Thrombocytopenic purpura and anemia in a breast-fed infant whose mother was treated with valproic acid. *J Pediatr* 1997;130: 1001–1003.

17 Steen B, Rane A, Lonnerholm G, Falk O, Elwin CE, Sjoqvist F. Phenytoin excretion in human breast milk and plasma levels in nursed infants. *Ther Drug Monit* 1982;4: 331–334.

18 Finch E, Lorber J. Methaemoglobinaemia in the newborn probably due to phenytoin excreted in human milk. *J Obstet Gynaecol Br Empire* 1954;61:833–834.

19 Shimoyama R, Ohkubo T, Sugawara K. Monitoring of carbamazepine and carbamazepine 10,11-epoxide in breast milk and plasma by high-performance liquid chromatography. *Ann Clin Biochem* 2000;37:210–215.

20 Froescher W, Eichelbaum M, Niesen M, Dietrich K, Rausch P. Carbamazepine levels in breast milk. *Ther Drug Monit* 1984;6:266–271.

21 Chaudron LH, Jefferson JW. Mood stabilizers during breastfeeding: a review. *J Clin Psychiatry* 2000;61:79–90.

22 Newport DJ, Pennell PB, Calamaras MR *et al.* Lamotrigine in breast milk and nursing infants: determination of exposure. *Pediatrics* 2008;122:e223–e231.

23 Fotopoulou C, Kretz R, Bauer S *et al.* Prospectively assessed changes in lamotrigine-concentration in women with epilepsy during pregnancy, lactation and the neonatal period. *Epilepsy Res* 2009;85:60–64.

24 Ohman I, Vitols S, Tomson T. Lamotrigine in pregnancy: pharmacokinetics during delivery, in the neonate, and during lactation. *Epilepsia* 2000;41:709–713.

25 Tomson T, Palm R, Kallen K *et al.* Pharmacokinetics of levetiracetam during pregnancy, delivery, in the neonatal period, and lactation. *Epilepsia* 2007;48:1111–1116.

26 Johannessen SI, Helde G, Brodtkorb E. Levetiracetam concentrations in serum and in breast milk at birth and during lactation. *Epilepsia* 2005;46:775–777.

27 Ohman I, Vitols S, Luef G, Soderfeldt B, Tomson T. Topiramate kinetics during delivery, lactation, and in the neonate: preliminary observations. *Epilepsia* 2002;43:1157–1160.

28 Kawada K, Itoh S, Kusaka T, Isobe K, Ishii M. Pharmacokinetics of zonisamide in perinatal period. *Brain Dev* 2002;24:95–97.
29 Bagshaw J, Crawford P, Chappell B. Problems that mothers' with epilepsy experience when caring for their children. *Seizure* 2008;17:42–48.
30 Pearlstein T, Howard M, Salisbury A, Zlotnick C. Postpartum depression. *Am J Obstet Gynecol* 2009;200:357–364.
31 Turner K, Piazzini A, Franza A *et al*. Postpartum depression in women with epilepsy versus women without epilepsy. *Epilepsy Behav* 2006;9:293–297.
32 Galanti M, Newport DJ, Pennell PB *et al*. Postpartum depression in women with epilepsy: influence of antiepileptic drugs in a prospective study. *Epilepsy Behav* 2009;16:426–430.

CHAPTER 17

Management of Epilepsy and Pregnancy

Sanjeev V. Thomas[1], Torbjörn Tomson[2] and Cynthia L. Harden[3]

[1]Department of Neurology, Sree Chitra Tirunal Institute for Medical Sciences and Technology, Trivandrum, Kerala, India

[2]Department of Clinical Neuroscience, Karolinska Institutet, Stockholm, Sweden

[3]North Shore-Long Island Jewish Health System, New York, USA

Forming a family is perhaps the most important aspect of life, for persons with epilepsy just as much as for anyone else. Although the vast majority of women with epilepsy can have uneventful pregnancies and give birth to perfectly normal children, some special considerations and precautions are justified. The importance and complexity of this issue is reflected in the fact that 12 chapters in this volume are dedicated to various aspects of epilepsy and reproductive health. These chapters provide updated separate reviews on fetal and maternal risks with seizures (Chapter 10), seizure control during pregnancy (Chapter 8), effects of pregnancy on antiepileptic drug (AED) disposition (Chapter 9), obstetrical outcome and complications (Chapter 11), mechanisms of teratogenic effects (Chapter 12), major congenital malformations (Chapter 13), fetal AED syndromes (Chapter 14), postnatal cognitive development (Chapter 15), and breastfeeding (Chapter 16). The challenge, however, is to synthesize these data into recommendations for the management of women with epilepsy during pregnancy. Despite the risk of teratogenic effects, physicians need to prescribe AEDs to women with active epilepsy who consider becoming pregnant, since uncontrolled seizures may harm the woman with epilepsy as well as her fetus. These risks need to balanced and a treatment has to be selected that is effective in preventing major seizures while at the same time minimizing adverse fetal drug effects.

Ambitious attempts have been made to develop evidence-based practice parameters for the management of women with epilepsy in pregnancy [1–3]. However, due to obvious ethical constraints, randomized studies are rare in this field and the evidence base thus weak and limited. Therefore, this short chapter summarizes in bullet points the editors'

Epilepsy in Women, First Edition. Edited by Cynthia L. Harden, Sanjeev V. Thomas and Torbjörn Tomson.
© 2013 John Wiley & Sons, Ltd. Published 2013 by John Wiley & Sons, Ltd.

expert consensus on the management of women with epilepsy during pregnancy. The reader is referred to the respective chapters for detailed background data. The editors, and authors of this short chapter, represent three continents, Asia, Europe and North America. We are thus fully aware of the need to adapt any recommendations to the local setting, taking into account cultural differences as well as disparities in resources and treatment traditions. To be relevant in this more global perspective, our recommendations focus on general principles and so lack detail somewhat. The recommendations are separated into actions to be considered prior to, during, and after pregnancy.

Prior to planning pregnancy

- Review current seizure frequency and severity. If seizures persist (in particular generalized tonic–clonic), consider further seizure management before endorsing pregnancy at this time. The potential teratogenic effects of AEDs need to be carefully weighed against the efficacy of the drug to control seizures. The relative cost difference between drugs is another important consideration in countries where the patients have to bear the treatment costs themselves. It is important to keep in mind that the overall risk of malformations is less than 10% if the woman is on monotherapy with relatively low dose (Chapter 13).
- If epilepsy is in remission, consider suggesting gradual withdrawal of treatment before pregnancy if recurrence risk is low and the woman willing to take the risk.
- Review history for congenital malformations with previous pregnancies or family history of such. Should this be present, discuss the higher risk of malformations, consider genetics consult, consider a switch from the AED used in previous pregnancy that resulted in malformations, and encourage more intensive monitoring in future pregnancy.
- Review current birth control and how it will be withdrawn before pregnancy.
- Review all medications. If the woman is taking valproate, change in medication should be considered. The nuances of selecting AEDs to treat women with epilepsy in the childbearing period are further discussed in Chapters 13 and 15.
- Review history for, or try out, lowest effective dose and, where this is possible to obtain, the corresponding level of the AED.
- If the woman is taking lowest effective dose of appropriate AED, obtain serum level preferably on two occasions weeks apart, and as trough level before morning dose. This is in order to obtain range of effective levels

and to assess stability of levels within the patient. If available obtain free and total levels if the AED is phenytoin or valproate (Chapters 8 and 9).
- Suggest that she takes 4–5 mg of folic acid per day.
- All changes in AED therapy should be completed and fully evaluated before conception.

During pregnancy

- Continue folic acid and prenatal vitamins throughout pregnancy.
- Avoid switches between AEDs unless prompted by poor maternal seizure control. A switch implies polytherapy exposure during the transition and also introduction of a new AED with unknown efficacy and tolerability in the individual woman. Avoid AED withdrawals during pregnancy because of the risk of seizure relapse and since the potential benefits for fetal exposure are questionable with the necessary slow tapering.
- Epilepsy that had been in remission may rarely relapse during pregnancy. Hormonal imbalance, other metabolic changes, or decrease in blood level of the AED may predispose to seizure exacerbation during pregnancy. More details of such variations are discussed in Chapter 8. Physicians need to have a plan to handle breakthrough seizures during pregnancy. Monitor for seizure occurrence regularly, frequency of contact depending on seizure control before and during pregnancy.
- Where methods are available, obtain serum AED levels at time of pregnancy confirmation and at regular intervals throughout pregnancy. In the case of carbamazepine and valproate this may be less frequent; in the case of lamotrigine, obtain levels monthly and consider increase in dose in a proportional manner to restore individual pre-pregnancy therapeutic level. Obtain free and total levels if the woman is taking phenytoin or valproate (Chapters 8 and 9).
- Monitor for vomiting of AEDs, and if it is occurring consider methods to reduce vomiting with assistance from obstetrician.
- Follow obstetrical outcomes, including ultrasound results. Suggest high-level ultrasound at 14–18 weeks for detailed view of fetal structures.
- If a malformation is recognized on ultrasonography, the pregnancy would require more detailed evaluation. Confirmatory tests such as fetal magnetic resonance imaging (MRI), amniocentesis, and other procedures are part of the evaluation in some regions. Further counseling on the possible impact of the suspected malformation on the health of the baby should be discussed by persons experienced in this field. The couple may require assistance in deciding on further course of action such as continuation or termination of pregnancy. Undue attribution of all complications to the use of AEDs or occurrence of seizures during pregnancy can lead to severe emotional and social stress and should be avoided.

- All seizures that occur during pregnancy may not be epilepsy. A variety of causes including eclampsia, acute symptomatic seizures, and new-onset epilepsy can manifest during pregnancy. A more detailed discussion on this is available in Chapter 4. A clinician should ascertain the type of epilepsy or seizure disorder as the treatment may differ according to the cause of seizures.
- If seizures occur late in pregnancy with therapeutic AED levels, monitor for preeclampsia and discuss delivery induction if appropriate.

After delivery

- If patient is stable and the dose has been increased during pregnancy, decrease AED dose over 10 days after delivery to a dose slightly above pre-pregnancy maintenance dose, to compensate for fatigue and postpartum sleep deprivation. A more rapid return to a lower dose may be needed for lamotrigine to avoid concentration-dependent adverse effects in the postpartum period.
- Encourage breastfeeding but indicate that adverse effects could occur occasionally if the mother is taking phenobarbital (Chapter 16).
- Counsel the patient about getting adequate sleep and to report adverse mood effects.
- Infant development is closely related to physical and behavioral stimulation of the infant. Mothers need to be encouraged to actively care for their babies, provide adequate nutritional and emotional support, and monitor their growth and development. Optimal contraception needs to be adopted to ensure adequate spacing between pregnancies (Chapter 16).

References

1 Harden CL, Hopp J, Ting TY *et al*. Management issues for women with epilepsy. Focus on pregnancy (an evidence-based review). I. Obstetrical complications and change in seizure frequency: Report of the Quality Standards Subcommittee and Therapeutics and Technology Assessment Subcommittee of the American Academy of Neurology and the American Epilepsy Society. *Epilepsia* 2009;50:1229–1236.
2 Harden CL, Meador KJ, Pennell PB *et al*. Management issues for women with epilepsy. Focus on pregnancy (an evidence-based review). II. Teratogenesis and perinatal outcomes: Report of the Quality Standards Subcommittee and Therapeutics and Technology Subcommittee of the American Academy of Neurology and the American Epilepsy Society. *Epilepsia* 2009;50:1237–1246.
3 Harden CL, Pennell PB, Koppel BS *et al*. Management issues for women with epilepsy. Focus on pregnancy (an evidence-based review). III. Vitamin K, folic acid, blood levels, and breast-feeding: Report of the Quality Standards Subcommittee and Therapeutics and Technology Assessment Subcommittee of the American Academy of Neurology and the American Epilepsy Society. *Epilepsia* 2009;50:1247–1255.

CHAPTER 18

Perimenopause and Menopause

Cynthia L. Harden

North Shore-Long Island Jewish Health System, New York, USA

> **Case history:** *A 49-year-old woman with a history of well-controlled complex partial seizures which began at age 24 reports a recent increase in seizure frequency. She had been stable with no seizures while taking carbamazepine for the previous 15 years. There is no known cause of seizures, and no risk factors for epilepsy including no history of head trauma, family members with epilepsy, or childhood developmental difficulties. Recent brain magnetic resonance imaging (MRI) is normal and EEG shows intermittent left temporal slowing. She is now having one seizure every 6–8 weeks, consisting of a brief confusional spell without associated injury. She rarely misses her twice-daily carbamazepine doses. She states that her last menstrual period was 4 months ago and that her menses have been irregular and scant for the past year. She also reports rare "hot flashes" that do not keep her awake at night.*

Background

Women with epilepsy face ongoing issues involving the interactions between their seizures, their reproductive life, and their treatments [1]. Perimenopause is another epoch during which epilepsy may destabilize, due to factors including the neuroexcitatory endogenous hormonal milieu of perimenopause, and difficulty sleeping from vasomotor activity. At menopause, for the first time since early childhood, women do not experience hormonal fluctuations; this stable endogenous hormonal state may also be stabilizing for seizure occurrence.

Perimenopause is characterized by decreased ovarian secretion of progesterone, resulting in increasing occurrence of anovulatory menstrual cycles. However, ovarian estrogen secretion remains robust until late perimenopause, and "surges" to high levels in the late luteal phase in approximately one-third of menstrual cycles during perimenopause [2,3]. Therefore, the perimenopausal neurosteroid environment is overall excitatory, with estrogen levels both maintained and even intermittently surging to high levels, but without the counterbalancing neuronal

Epilepsy in Women, First Edition. Edited by Cynthia L. Harden, Sanjeev V. Thomas and Torbjörn Tomson.
© 2013 John Wiley & Sons, Ltd. Published 2013 by John Wiley & Sons, Ltd.

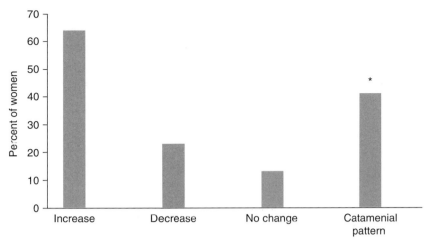

Figure 18.1 Perimenopausal women: epilepsy pattern. *, Significantly associated with increase in seizures ($P=0.02$). HRT significantly associated with increase in seizures ($P=0.001$). (From Harden CL, Pulver MC, Jacobs AR. The effect of menopause and perimenopause on the course of epilepsy. *Epilepsia* 1999;40:1402–1407 with permission.)

inhibitory effects of progesterone metabolites. The increased estrogen secretion at perimenopause, due to follicle-stimulating hormone (FSH), eventually diminishes, producing the hypogonadal state of menopause [3]. This hypothalamic–pituitary–gonadal hormonal shift would predictably be associated with an increase in seizure occurrence at perimenopause, although this aspect of the experiences of women with epilepsy has been little studied.

One cross-sectional evaluation on the course of epilepsy through the perimenopause and menopausal transition was gathered from mailed questionnaires to a large group of women in an epilepsy specialty practice as well as women from a local epilepsy advocacy organization database [4]. Almost two-thirds of perimenopausal women with epilepsy, defined as recent onset of menstrual changes or "hot flashes," reported an increase in seizures during perimenopause. A history of a catamenial seizure pattern, defined as increased seizures in the week before the onset of menses, was significantly associated with an increase in seizure frequency at perimenopause (Figure 18.1) [4]. Women who were menopausal, defined as 1 year without menses, reported no overall directional change in seizure frequency at menopause; approximately one-third each reported an increase, decrease, or no change in seizure frequency after becoming menopausal.

The finding of no overall directional change in seizure frequency at menopause is consistent with a previous report [5,6]. However, a history of a catamenial seizure pattern in the questionnaire menopausal group correlated with reporting a decrease in seizure frequency at menopause [4]. These findings support the concept that a subset of women with epilepsy are sensitive to endogenous hormonal changes during reproductive years and as these years wane. Further, a high percentage of women in the perimenopause group in this study took synthetic hormone replacement therapy (HRT), which was significantly associated with an increase in seizures ($P=0.001$) [4].

Because of the HRT association found, this questionnaire study was followed up with a randomized, double-blind, placebo-controlled trial of HRT in menopausal women with epilepsy in order to prospectively study the effect of HRT on seizure frequency [7]. The interventions used were as follows: 0.625 mg of conjugated equine estrogens plus 2.5 mg of medroxyprogesterone acetate (CEE/MPA; brand name Prempro) at either single dose or double dose daily, or placebo, used for 3 months following a prospective baseline period. After randomizing only a small number of subjects (due to the report of increased rates of breast cancer associated with this form of HRT), the investigators found that seizure frequency significantly increased with the use of CEE/MPA in a dose-related manner [7]. In general, HRT is now used less frequently due to associated health risks, although it may have a role in the transition for some women [8]. For women with epilepsy, the clinical trial findings provide evidence against the use of CEE/MPA because of seizure risks and, importantly, demonstrate that exogenous reproductive hormones can have predictable clinical effects on persons with epilepsy.

Women with epilepsy are also at risk for early onset of ovarian failure, which translates clinically as the menopausal transition. The mechanism is likely related to hypothalamic–pituitary–gonadal axis dysfunction, producing dysregulation of maturation of ovarian follicles and early loss of follicles available for ovulation. In the first report of early perimenopause in women with epilepsy [9], 14% of women with epilepsy had premature ovarian failure compared with 3.7% of healthy control women ($P-0.04$). Additionally, women with premature ovarian failure were more likely to have had catamenial exacerbation of their seizures during earlier reproductive years. It has also been reported that the risk for earlier menopause may be related to seizure frequency. In this study, a negative correlation was found between age at menopause and seizure frequency ($P=0.014$) [10]. For example, the women with only rare seizures had a normal age at menopause of 50–51 years, while women with frequent seizures experienced earlier menopause at 46–47 years [10]. Conceptually, if epilepsy is itself an endocrine disruptor, more frequent seizures would confer a more severe dose effect.

Implications for management

The implications for management during perimenopause and menopause generally encompass having an understanding of the patient in terms of her history of catamenial seizure patterns, ongoing reproductive state, and whether vasomotor symptoms are interfering with sleep, since this may be an important factor for seizure increase as well [11]. Management should include increased vigilance for seizure occurrence at perimenopause, and a low threshold for relieving vasomotor symptoms that interfere with sleep, although not with the use of CEE/MPA. Seizure freedom is always a goal of treatment, and for women with epilepsy this may prolong the period of reproductive years to a normal duration.

Review of the case: *The patient is clearly perimenopausal and likely experiencing more seizures due to the associated hormonal changes. Her carbamazepine levels were checked and found to be in her usual range, which was therapeutic but less than 7 µg/mL. Her dose was increased by 25% and seizures did not recur. After she became menopausal 18 months later without seizure recurrence, the carbamazepine dose was decreased back to the original dose with no problems. She had occasional "hot flashes" and the use of estradiol with natural progesterone lozenges was discussed. However, her sleep was not disrupted and the events were infrequent. Therefore, in consultation with her gynecologist, no intervention was undertaken.*

 Key summary points

- Understand if the patient has had a catamenial seizure pattern; this may be particularly associated with increased seizures at perimenopause.

- Query the patient for her reproductive status and monitor for increased seizures at perimenopause. Check levels of appropriate AEDs and consider maintaining higher therapeutic levels.

- Advise perimenopausal patients to be vigilant with taking AEDs and getting adequate sleep.

- If vasomotor symptoms disrupt sleep, do not use CEE/MPA to relieve them, but consult with a gynecologist for other treatment approaches.

References

1 Prior JC, Hitchcock CL. The endocrinology of perimenopause: need for a paradigm shift. *Front Biosci (Schol Ed)* 2011;3:474–486.
2 Burger HG, Dudley EC, Robertson DM, Dennerstein L. Hormonal changes in the menopause transition. *Recent Prog Horm Res* 2002;57:257–275.
3 Burger HG. Diagnostic role of follicle stimulating hormone (FSH) measurements during menopausal transition: an analysis of FSH, oestradiol and inhibin. *Eur J Endocrinol* 1994;130:38–42.
4 Harden CL, Pulver MC, Jacobs AR. The effect of menopause and perimenopause on the course of epilepsy. *Epilepsia* 1999;40:1402–1407.

5 Abbasi F, Krumholz A, Kittner SJ, Langenberg P. Effects of menopause on seizures in women with epilepsy. *Epilepsia* 1999;40:205–210.

6 McAuley JW, Koshy SJ, Moore JL, Peebles CT, Reeves AL. Characterization and health risk assessment of postmenopausal women with epilepsy. *Epilepsy Behav* 2000;1:353–355.

7 Harden CL, Herzog AG, Nikolov BG *et al*. Hormone replacement therapy in WWE: a randomized, double-blind, placebo-controlled study. *Epilepsia* 2006;47:1447–1451.

8 North American Menopause Society. Estrogen and progestogen use in postmenopausal women: 2010 position statement of the North American Menopause Society. *Menopause* 2010;17:242–55.

9 Klein P, Serje A, Pezzullo JC. Premature ovarian failure in WWE. *Epilepsia* 2001;42:1584–1589.

10 Harden CL, Koppel BS, Herzog AG, Nikolov BG, Hauser WA. Seizure frequency is associated with age of menopause in WWE. *Neurology* 2003;61:451–455.

11 Peebles CT, McAuley JW, Moore JL, Malone HJ, Reeves AL. Hormone replacement therapy in a postmenopausal woman with epilepsy. *Ann Pharmacother* 2000;34: 1028–1031.

CHAPTER 19

Bone Health

Alison M. Pack

Department of Neurology, Neurological Institute of New York, Columbia University Medical Center, New York, USA

Case history: S.G. is a 59-year-old woman with a history of primary generalized epilepsy diagnosed at age 11. She initially presented with "petit mal" or absence seizures. She has not had an absence seizure since she was a teenager. She later began having generalized tonic–clonic seizures. She has had less than 10 generalized tonic–clonic seizures throughout her life; the last one occurred over 20 years ago. She was treated with phenytoin and phenobarbital and has taken this combination of medications for over 40 years. She had her first bone mineral density (BMD) dual energy-X ray absorptiometry (DXA) scan 4 years ago revealing osteoporosis at multiple sites: total hip (T-score –3.3), femoral neck of the hip (T-score –3.6), and lumbar spine (T-score –2.8). Osteoporosis in postmenopausal women is defined as having T-scores less than –2.5. Other than being postmenopausal (menopause occurred at age 49) and prolonged use of phenytoin and phenobarbital, she has no other risk factors for osteoporosis. She has no significant history of alcohol or tobacco use, family history of osteoporosis, and has never taken glucocorticosteroids. After she was diagnosed with having osteoporosis, she was treated with the antiresorptive agent alendronate for 3 years. Despite taking this agent, she continued to lose bone mass at all sites. More recently she is being treated with teriparatide and was transitioned off phenytoin.

Background

Persons with epilepsy treated with antiepileptic drugs (AEDs) are at increased risk for poor bone health including increased risk of fracture, low BMD, and abnormalities in bone and mineral metabolism. Studies support abnormalities in bone health in association with both epilepsy and AED exposure. Cytochrome P450-inducing AEDs are most consistently associated with adverse effects on bone.

The risk of fracture among children and adults with epilepsy is two to six times greater than in the general population [1,2]. Multiple factors including propensity to fall, seizures, and AED exposure contribute

---

Epilepsy in Women, First Edition. Edited by Cynthia L. Harden, Sanjeev V. Thomas and Torbjörn Tomson.

to the increased risk. Persons with epilepsy may fall during a seizure, particularly a generalized tonic–clonic seizure, and subsequently increase the risk of fracture. In support of this concept, generalized tonic–clonic seizures are associated with a higher risk for fracture than partial seizures [3].

AED exposure independently increases fracture risk. Multiple population-based studies in the UK [4], Denmark [5], and the USA [6] find a positive association between AED use and fracture. AED exposure may influence fracture risk by impacting balance. In a study of 29 ambulatory community-dwelling twin and sibling pairs discordant for AED use, balance performance was found to be impaired among the AED users [7]. Increased duration of AED exposure and AED polytherapy were independent predictors of balance impairment.

Individual AEDs differentially affect fracture risk. In a Danish pharmaco-epidemiologic population-based case-control study, after adjusting for significant confounders including a diagnosis of epilepsy, carbamazepine, clonazepam, phenobarbital, and valproate were all associated with a significant increase in fracture risk [8]. Other studies suggest that cytochrome P450-inducing AEDs independently increase the risk of fracture [6,8].

BMD is a significant predictor of fracture and studies find low BMD in 38–60% of persons with epilepsy treated with AEDs [9–11]. Longer AED use is associated with decreased BMD [9,10,12]. Children as well as adults with epilepsy treated with AEDs have low BMD [12–16]. The findings in children are relevant as childhood and adolescence are important periods of bone accrual; therefore the lower BMD reported in children with epilepsy treated with AEDs suggests that these children may have abnormal bone mineralization and development during this critical period.

As with fracture risk, AEDs differentially affect BMD [1,17,18]. Cytochrome P450-inducing AEDs including phenytoin and phenobarbital are most consistently associated with low BMD [1,17–21]. Although carbamazepine is a cytochrome P450-inducing AED, studies are not as consistent when looking at an association between carbamazepine and low BMD [9,12,14–16,19,22–24]. As with carbamazepine, findings regarding the effect of valproate on BMD are mixed [11,12,14,16,19,24]. Although one study found reduced BMD in children treated with lamotrigine, the findings most closely correlated with reduced exercise [25]. Other adult and pediatric studies do not find reduced BMD in association with lamotrigine treatment [19,26]. Among other commonly used AEDs the effect of gabapentin, oxcarbazepine and topiramate on BMD has been studied. Studies including gabapentin find that long-term gabapentin results in bone loss at both the hip and spine [22,27,28]. Two 1-year prospective studies assessed the relationship between oxcarbazepine and BMD and found no significant BMD loss in 28 adults [29] and in 34 pediatric newly diagnosed subjects [30]. Topiramate treatment in 36 women was not associated with any difference in BMD when compared with a control group of women or women treated with carbamazepine and valproate [31].

Persons with epilepsy treated with AEDs are at risk for abnormalities in bone and mineral metabolism. These abnormalities can predispose to reduced BMD and fracture. Studies suggest that persons with epilepsy are not getting enough calcium [32]. Active vitamin D metabolites, notably 25-hydroxyvitamin D, may be low in persons with epilepsy [1,18]. However, this is not a consistent finding. When reported, enzyme-inducing AEDs are most commonly associated with lower levels of 25-hydroxyvitamin D [1,18]. Bone turnover markers are measurements of bone formation and bone resorption. Elevated bone turnover markers reflect increased bone remodeling, are associated with higher rates of bone loss, and are independent predictors of fracture. Elevations in bone formation and resorption markers have been reported with AED therapy [1,18,33–36].

Implications for management

Poor bone health can occur as a consequence of epilepsy as well as AED therapy. When treating a person with epilepsy, one should consider factors that would predispose a patient to develop adverse effects on bone, particularly fracture. Optimizing seizure control, particularly reducing generalized tonic–clonic seizures, and minimizing AED effects on balance will reduce the propensity for the patient to fall. The specific chosen AED may have a long-term negative impact on bone health. For example, cytochrome P450-inducing AEDs are most commonly associated with increased risk of fracture, low BMD, and abnormalities in bone and mineral metabolism. Monitoring of calcium and vitamin D metabolites is important as some AEDs may affect their concentrations. Current guidelines suggest that 25-hydroxyvitamin D concentrations should be above 30 ng/mL. Enzyme-inducing AEDs may require a higher dose of vitamin D supplementation in order to achieve an adequate concentration of 25-hydroxyvitamin D. DXA scanning should be considered in those at risk for low BMD, particularly in persons with multiple risk factors for low BMD and fracture (e.g., family history of epilepsy, glucocorticosteroid use). For those with low BMD, multiple therapeutic agents are available. If a person is taking an AED known to result in adverse effects on bone, changing that AED may improve bone health.

> **Review of the case:** *S.G. is a postmenopausal woman who was treated for over 40 years with two cytochrome P450-inducing AEDs known to negatively affect bone health. Other than being menopausal, she had no other risk factors for reduced BMD. DXA scans revealed osteoporosis at multiple sites, significantly increasing her risk of fracture. As well, she was taking AEDs that may affect balance and increase her propensity to fall. She was treated with a bisphosphonate, but continued to lose bone mass. In reviewing her history, consideration should have been given years ago to the impact of the chosen AEDs on bone health. The patient was not aware that the AEDs she was taking may have affected her bones. She never had screening of 25-hydroxyvitamin D and did not get a DXA scan until 6 years after menopause. By then she had significant bone loss or osteoporosis at multiple sites. Following failure of bisphosphonate therapy, she was treated with teriparatide and was transitioned off phenytoin. Her BMD has improved at all sites.*

 Key summary points

- Having epilepsy as well as AED treatment can negatively impact bone health.
- Persons with epilepsy have a twofold to sixfold increased risk of fracture.
- Generalized tonic–clonic seizures and impaired balance may increase one's risk of falling and sustaining a fracture.
- AED treatment is associated with increased risk of fracture, low BMD, and abnormalities in bone and mineral metabolism. Cytochrome P450-inducing AEDs including phenytoin and phenobarbital are most consistently associated with adverse effects on bone.

References

1 Pack AM. Treatment of epilepsy to optimize bone health. *Curr Treat Options Neurol* 2011;13:346–354.
2 Souverein PC, Webb DJ, Petri H, Weil J, Van Staa TP, Egberts T. Incidence of fractures among epilepsy patients: a population-based retrospective cohort study in the General Practice Research Database. *Epilepsia* 2005;46:304–310.
3 Persson HB, Alberts KA, Farahmand BY, Tomson T. Risk of extremity fractures in adult outpatients with epilepsy. *Epilepsia* 2002;43:768–772.
4 Souverein PC, Webb DJ, Weil JG, Van Staa TP, Egberts AC. Use of antiepileptic drugs and risk of fractures: case–control study among patients with epilepsy. *Neurology* 2006;66:1318–1324.
5 Tsiropoulos I, Andersen M, Nymark T, Lauritsen J, Gaist D, Hallas J. Exposure to antiepileptic drugs and the risk of hip fracture: a case–control study. *Epilepsia* 2008;49: 2092–2099.
6 Carbone LD, Johnson KC, Robbins J *et al.* Antiepileptic drug use, falls, fractures, and BMD in postmenopausal women: findings from the women's health initiative (WHI). *J Bone Miner Res* 2010;25:873–881.
7 Petty SJ, Hill KD, Haber NE *et al.* Balance impairment in chronic antiepileptic drug users: a twin and sibling study. *Epilepsia* 2010;51:280–288.

8 Vestergaard P, Rejnmark L, Mosekilde L. Fracture risk associated with use of antiepileptic drugs. *Epilepsia* 2004;45:1330–1337.

9 Andress DL, Ozuna J, Tirschwell D *et al*. Antiepileptic drug-induced bone loss in young male patients who have seizures. *Arch Neurol* 2002;59:781–786.

10 Farhat G, Yamout B, Mikati MA, Demirjian S, Sawaya R, El-Hajj Fuleihan G. Effect of antiepileptic drugs on bone density in ambulatory patients. *Neurology* 2002;58:1348–1353.

11 Sato Y, Kondo I, Ishida S *et al*. Decreased bone mass and increased bone turnover with valproate therapy in adults with epilepsy. *Neurology* 2001;57:445–449.

12 Sheth RD, Wesolowski CA, Jacob JC *et al*. Effect of carbamazepine and valproate on bone mineral density. *J Pediatr* 1995;127:256–262.

13 Sheth RD, Gidal BE, Hermann BP. Pathological fractures in epilepsy. *Epilepsy Behav* 2006;9:601–605.

14 Erbayat Altay E, Serdaroglu A, Tumer L, Gucuyener K, Hasanoglu A. Evaluation of bone mineral metabolism in children receiving carbamazepine and valproic acid. *J Pediatr Endocrinol Metab* 2000;13:933–939.

15 Tekgul H, Serdaroglu G, Huseyinov A, Gokben S. Bone mineral status in pediatric outpatients on antiepileptic drug monotherapy. *J Child Neurol* 2006;21:411–414.

16 Kumandas S, Koklu E, Gumus H *et al*. Effect of carbamazepine and valproic acid on bone mineral density, IGF-I and IGFBP-3. *J Pediatr Endocrinol Metab* 2006;19:529–534.

17 Verrotti A, Coppola G, Parisi P, Mohn A, Chiarelli F. Bone and calcium metabolism and antiepileptic drugs. *Clin Neurol Neurosurg* 2010;112:1–10.

18 Pack AM, Walczak TS. Bone health in women with epilepsy: clinical features and potential mechanisms. *Int Rev Neurobiol* 2008;83:305–328.

19 Pack AM, Morrell MJ, Randall A, McMahon DJ, Shane E. Bone health in young women with epilepsy after one year of antiepileptic drug monotherapy. *Neurology* 2008;70:1586–1593.

20 Valimaki MJ, Tiihonen M, Laitinen K *et al*. Bone mineral density measured by dual-energy x-ray absorptiometry and novel markers of bone formation and resorption in patients on antiepileptic drugs. *J Bone Miner Res* 1994;9:631–637.

21 Stephen LJ, McLellan AR, Harrison JH *et al*. Bone density and antiepileptic drugs: a case-controlled study. *Seizure* 1999;8:339–342.

22 El-Hajj Fuleihan G, Dib L, Yamout B, Sawaya R, Mikati MA. Predictors of bone density in ambulatory patients on antiepileptic drugs. *Bone* 2008;43:149–155.

23 Kafali G, Erselcan T, Tanzer F. Effect of antiepileptic drugs on bone mineral density in children between ages 6 and 12 years. *Clin Pediatr (Phila)* 1999;38:93–98.

24 Kim SH, Lee JW, Choi KG, Chung HW, Lee HW. A 6-month longitudinal study of bone mineral density with antiepileptic drug monotherapy. *Epilepsy Behav* 2007;10:291–295.

25 Guo CY, Ronen GM, Atkinson SA. Long-term valproate and lamotrigine treatment may be a marker for reduced growth and bone mass in children with epilepsy. *Epilepsia* 2001;42:1141–1147.

26 Sheth RD, Hermann BP. Bone mineral density with lamotrigine monotherapy for epilepsy. *Pediatr Neurol* 2007;37:250–254.

27 Vestergaard P, Rejnmark L, Mosekilde L. Anxiolytics and sedatives and risk of fractures: effects of half-life. *Calcif Tissue Int* 2008;82:34–43.

28 Ensrud KE, Walczak TS, Blackwell TL, Ensrud ER, Barrett-Connor E, Orwoll ES. Antiepileptic drug use and rates of hip bone loss in older men: a prospective study. *Neurology* 2008;71:723–730.

29 Cetinkaya Y, Kurtulmus YS, Tutkavul K, Tireli H. The effect of oxcarbazepine on bone metabolism. *Acta Neurol Scand* 2009;120:170–175.

30 Cansu A, Yesilkaya E, Serdaroglu A *et al*. Evaluation of bone turnover in epileptic children using oxcarbazepine. *Pediatr Neurol* 2008;39:266–271.

31 Heo K, Rhee Y, Lee HW *et al*. The effect of topiramate monotherapy on bone mineral density and markers of bone and mineral metabolism in premenopausal women with epilepsy. *Epilepsia* 2011;52:1884–1889.

32 Menon B, Harinarayan CV, Raj MN, Vemuri S, Himabindu G, Afsana TK. Prevalence of low dietary calcium intake in patients with epilepsy: a study from South India. *Neurol India* 2010;58:209–212.

33 Samaniego EA, Sheth RD. Bone consequences of epilepsy and antiepileptic medications. *Semin Pediatr Neurol* 2007;14:196–200.

34 Verrotti A, Greco R, Morgese G, Chiarelli F. Increased bone turnover in epileptic patients treated with carbamazepine. *Ann Neurol* 2000;47:385–388.

35 Verrotti A, Greco R, Latini G, Morgese G, Chiarelli F. Increased bone turnover in pre-pubertal, pubertal, and postpubertal patients receiving carbamazepine. *Epilepsia* 2002;43:1488–1492.

36 Verrotti A, Agostinelli S, Coppola G, Parisi P, Chiarelli F. A 12-month longitudinal study of calcium metabolism and bone turnover during valproate monotherapy. *Eur J Neurol* 2010;17:232–237.

Index

Note: Page references in *italics* refer to Figures; those in **bold** refer to Tables

---

Epilepsy in Women, First Edition. Edited by Cynthia L. Harden, Sanjeev V. Thomas
and Torbjörn Tomson.
© 2013 John Wiley & Sons, Ltd. Published 2013 by John Wiley & Sons, Ltd.